Fat Burning Basics

If you're overweight, you are not a bad person. You're simply overweight. But it's important to lose the extra pounds so you'll look good, feel healthier, and develop a sense of pride and self-esteem. Once you've lost the fat, you'll need to maintain your weight.

In this booklet, you'll discover how to lose 10 pounds a month – a nice, safe loss of about two or two-and-a-half pounds a week – painlessly. You'll feel satisfied and more energetic than in the past without feeling deprived.

Most Americans pack on those extra pounds by eating the wrong things. Changing these poor eating habits is the key to long-term success. Knowledge – along with the right food – is the key.

When humans lived in caves, they didn't know anything about preserving and storing food. They spent all their waking time and energy hunting and gathering food. When they had it, they gobbled it down fast. Instead of storing food in pantries or cupboards, they stored energy in their bodies in the form of fat to burn during periods when there was little or nothing to eat.

Each year, it was vital for them to put on a good layer of fat during the warm sprint and summer months. That was the only way they could guarantee their survival during the lean and mean winter months.

And since women bore the young, they needed more energy to sustain themselves and their babies, and that meant they were usually heavier.

Even though we no longer live in caves, we have inherited and maintained this basic mechanism for fat storage from our hunting and gathering ancestors.

Each one of us is born with a certain number of fat cells. How many of these fat cells you possess depends on genetics. If you have a lot of fat cells, maybe your ancestors were the biggest people in the tribe, which was a good thing because they had the best chances of survival.

You can never get rid of fat cells, but – unfortunately – you can add to them. Depending upon what you eat, your body will manufacture new far cells. And like those you were born with, they never go away.

That doesn't mean you're doomed to be fat once you put on extra pounds. It is possible to shrink fat cells. That's what happens when you lose weight. You burn up the fat stored in those big fat cells. Think of them as balloons. Burning off the fat inside them has the same effect as letting the air out of a balloon.

A good weight loss program requires a certain amount of intake restriction – the consumption of fewer calories. You burn off the fat by eating less fat and becoming more active.

To guarantee a lifetime of weight-control success, you have to change the type of foods you eat so that you ingest less fat and still get the vitamins, minerals, trace elements, protein, fat, and carbohydrates your body needs to thrive.

Extremely low-calorie diets may help you shed pounds quickly, but they'll lead to failure in the long run.

That's because humans are genetically protected against starvation. During food shortages, our bodies slow down our metabolisms and burn less energy so we can stay alive.

A part of our brain called the hypothalamus keeps us on an even weight by creating a "set point." That's the weight where we feel comfortable. The hypothalamus determines this point based on the level of consumption it's used to. It seeks to keep our weight constant, even if that point is over what it should be.

When we drastically cut back our food intake, the brain thinks the body is starving, and to preserve life, it slows the metabolism. Soon the pounds stop coming off. Consequently, we grow hungry and uncomfortable and then eat more. And then the diet fails.

How can you compensate for this metabolic slow-down? The answer is that you have to change the nutritional composition of the foods you eat. You will have to cut down on total calories – that's basic to weight loss. More important, however, is reducing the percentage of total calories you are getting from fat.

That's how you'll avoid starvation panic in your system. At the same time, you reduce the amount of fat in your food, replacing it with safe, low-calorie, nutrient-rich plant foods. This will convince your brain that your body is getting all the nutrition it needs.

You'll be able to eat more food and feel more satisfied while consuming fewer calories and fats.

Plant foods break down slowly in your stomach, making you feel full longer, and they are rich in vitamins, minerals, trace elements, carbohydrates, and protein for energy and muscle-building. This allows your body to burn off its excess stored fat.

Fat Burning Foods

Each one of the following foods is clinically proven to promote weight loss. These foods go a step beyond simply adding no fat to your system – they possess special properties that add zip to your system and help your body melt away unhealthy pounds. These incredible foods can suppress your appetite for junk food and keep your body running smoothly with clean fuel and efficient energy.

You can include these foods in any sensible weight-loss plan. They give your body the extra metabolic kick that it needs to shave off weight quickly.

A sensible weight loss plan calls for no fewer than 1,200 calories per day. But Dr. Charles Klein recommends consuming more than that, if you can believe it – 1,500 to 1,800 calories per day. He says you will still lose weight quite effectively at that intake level without endangering your health.

Hunger is satisfied more completely by filling the stomach. Ounce for ounce, the foods listed below accomplish that better than any others. At the same time, they're rich in nutrients and possess special fat-melting talents.

Apples

These marvels of nature deserve their reputation for keeping the doctor away when you eat one a day. And now, it seems, they can help you melt the fat away, too.

First of all, they elevate your blood glucose (sugar) levels in a safe, gentle manner and keep them up longer than most foods. The practical effect of this is to leave you feeling satisfied longer, say researchers.

Secondly, they're one of the richest sources of soluble fiber in the supermarket. This type of fiber prevents hunger pangs by guarding against dangerous swings or drops in your blood sugar level, says Dr. James Anderson of the University of Kentucky's School of Medicine.

An average-sized apple provides only 81 calories and has no sodium, saturated fat, or cholesterol. You'll also get the added health benefits of lowering the level of cholesterol already in your blood as well as lowering your blood pressure.

Apples, the quintessential fruit of fall, have long been celebrated for their crisp texture, refreshing flavor, and numerous health benefits. From ancient folklore to modern scientific research, the apple's reputation as a symbol of health and vitality is deeply ingrained in cultures worldwide. In this comprehensive exploration, we delve into the multifaceted benefits of apples, ranging from their nutritional composition to their potential impacts on various aspects of human health.

Nutritional Composition:

At the core of the apple's nutritional prowess lies its rich and diverse composition of vitamins, minerals, antioxidants, and dietary fiber. A medium-sized apple (approximately 182 grams) typically contains:

Calories: Around 95 calories, making it a low-calorie yet satisfying snack option.

Carbohydrates: Primarily in the form of natural sugars, including fructose, glucose, and sucrose.

Fiber: A notable source of dietary fiber, with an average apple providing approximately 4 grams, including both soluble and insoluble fiber.

Vitamins: Apples are a good source of vitamin C, providing about 14% of the recommended daily intake. They also contain small amounts of other vitamins, including vitamin A, vitamin K, and various B vitamins.

Minerals: While apples are not exceptionally rich in minerals, they do contain small amounts of potassium, manganese, and other trace minerals.

Antioxidants: Apples are rich in various phytochemicals, including flavonoids, polyphenols, and quercetin, which possess antioxidant properties that help protect cells from oxidative damage.

Health Benefits:

Weight Management:

Apples are often touted as a weight-loss-friendly food due to their low calorie and high fiber content. The fiber in apples promotes satiety, reducing hunger and aiding in portion control.

Studies suggest that incorporating apples into a balanced diet may contribute to weight loss and improve overall body composition.

Heart Health:

Regular consumption of apples has been linked to a reduced risk of cardiovascular disease. The soluble fiber in apples helps lower LDL (bad) cholesterol levels, while the antioxidants help protect against oxidative stress and inflammation.

Potassium, another essential nutrient found in apples, supports heart health by regulating blood pressure and reducing the risk of hypertension.

Blood Sugar Control:

Despite their natural sugar content, apples have a low glycemic index, meaning they cause a gradual rise in blood sugar levels rather than a sharp spike.

The soluble fiber in apples slows down the absorption of glucose, helping to stabilize blood sugar levels and reduce the risk of insulin resistance and type 2 diabetes.

Digestive Health:

The fiber content in apples supports digestive health by promoting regular bowel movements and preventing constipation. Insoluble fiber adds bulk to stool, while soluble fiber nourishes beneficial gut bacteria.

Pectin, a type of soluble fiber found in apples, acts as a prebiotic, feeding the probiotic bacteria in the gut and promoting a healthy microbiome.

Cancer Prevention:

Some research suggests that the antioxidants and phytochemicals in apples may help reduce the risk of certain types of cancer, including colorectal cancer, due to their ability to neutralize free radicals and inhibit tumor growth.

Quercetin, a flavonoid abundant in apples, has been studied for its potential anti-cancer properties, although more research is needed to confirm these effects.

Brain Health:

Preliminary studies indicate that regular apple consumption may have cognitive benefits, including a reduced risk of neurodegenerative diseases such as Alzheimer's disease.

Antioxidants in apples help protect brain cells from oxidative stress and inflammation, which are implicated in age-related cognitive decline.

Respiratory Health:

Some evidence suggests that apples may have a protective effect against respiratory conditions such as asthma and chronic obstructive pulmonary disease (COPD). Quercetin, in particular, has been studied for its potential anti-inflammatory and bronchodilator effects.

Conclusion:

Apples, with their delicious flavor, crisp texture, and abundant health benefits, truly live up to their reputation as nature's nutritional powerhouse. From weight management to heart health, and digestive support to cancer prevention, the humble apple offers a wide array of benefits that contribute to overall well-being. Whether enjoyed fresh, baked into pies, or blended into smoothies, incorporating apples into a balanced diet is a simple yet effective way to enhance health and vitality. As we continue to unravel the mysteries of nutrition and health, the enduring appeal of the apple remains a testament to the enduring wisdom of nature's bounty.

Whole Grain Bread

You needn't dread bread. It's the butter, margarine, or cream cheese you put on it that's fattening, not the bread itself. We'll say this as often as needed – fat is fattening. If you don't believe that, ponder this – a gram of carbohydrate has four calories, a gram of protein four, and a gram of fat nine. So which of these is fattening?

Bread, a natural source of fiber and complex carbohydrates, is okay for dieting. Norwegian scientist Dr. Bjarne Jacobsen found that people who eat less than two slices of bread daily weigh about 11 pounds more that those who eat a lot of bread.

Studies at Michigan State University show some breads reduce the appetite. Researchers compared white bread to dark, high-fiber bread and found that students who ate 12 slices a day of the dark, high-fiber bread felt less hunger daily and lost five pounds in two months. Others who ate white bread were hungrier, ate more fattening foods, and lost no weight during this time.

So the key is eating dark, rich, high-fiber bread such as pumpernickel, whole wheat, mixed grain, oatmeal, and others. The average slice of whole grain bread contains only 60 to 70 calories, is rich in complex carbohydrates – the best, steadiest fuel you can give your body – and delivers a surprising amount of protein.

Nutritional Composition:

Whole grain bread derives its nutritional prowess from the intact grain kernel, comprising three key components: the bran, germ, and endosperm. This holistic composition provides a diverse array of essential nutrients, including:

Fiber:

Whole grain bread is an excellent source of dietary fiber, offering both soluble and insoluble fiber. Soluble fiber forms a gel-like substance in the digestive tract, helping to lower cholesterol levels and regulate blood sugar levels. Insoluble fiber adds bulk to stool, promoting regular bowel movements and supporting digestive health.

Vitamins and Minerals:

Whole grain bread contains a variety of vitamins and minerals, including B vitamins (such as thiamine, riboflavin, niacin, and folate), vitamin E, magnesium, iron, and zinc. These nutrients play vital roles in energy metabolism, immune function, and overall health.

Phytonutrients:

Whole grains are rich in phytonutrients, including antioxidants such as phenolic acids, flavonoids, and lignans. These compounds help neutralize free radicals, reduce inflammation, and protect against chronic diseases such as heart disease, cancer, and diabetes.

Health Benefits:

Heart Health:

Numerous studies have linked the consumption of whole grains, including whole grain bread, to a reduced risk of heart disease. The fiber, antioxidants, and phytonutrients in whole grains help lower cholesterol levels, reduce blood pressure, and improve overall cardiovascular health.

Whole grains also contain compounds like plant sterols and stanols, which inhibit the absorption of cholesterol in the intestine, further contributing to heart health.

Weight Management:

Whole grain bread's high fiber content promotes satiety and helps control appetite, making it a valuable component of a weight management plan. Studies have shown that individuals who consume more whole grains tend to have lower body weight and reduced risk of obesity.

The complex carbohydrates in whole grain bread provide sustained energy, preventing rapid spikes and crashes in blood sugar levels and supporting stable energy levels throughout the day.

Blood Sugar Control:

Unlike refined grains, which are quickly digested and absorbed, whole grains are digested more slowly, resulting in a gradual release of glucose into the bloodstream. This slower digestion helps regulate blood sugar levels and reduce the risk of insulin resistance and type 2 diabetes.

The fiber and magnesium content of whole grain bread further contributes to improved insulin sensitivity and blood sugar control.

Digestive Health:

The fiber-rich nature of whole grain bread promotes digestive health by supporting regular bowel movements, preventing constipation, and reducing the risk of diverticular disease.

Fermentable fibers in whole grains serve as prebiotics, nourishing beneficial gut bacteria and promoting a healthy microbiome, which is essential for overall digestive function and immune health.

Cancer Prevention:

Some research suggests that the antioxidants and phytonutrients in whole grains may help reduce the risk of certain types of cancer, including colorectal cancer. These compounds have been shown to inhibit cancer cell growth, induce apoptosis (cell death), and prevent the formation of tumors.

The fiber in whole grains may also help lower circulating levels of estrogen, which is associated with a reduced risk of hormone-related cancers such as breast and endometrial cancer.

Cognitive Health:

Emerging evidence suggests that whole grain consumption may be beneficial for cognitive function and brain health. The antioxidants and anti-inflammatory compounds in whole grains help protect brain cells from oxidative stress and inflammation, which are implicated in age-related cognitive decline and neurodegenerative diseases such as Alzheimer's disease.

Coffee

Easy does it is the password here. We've all heard about potential dangers of caffeine – including anxiety and insomnia – so moderation is the key.

The caffeine in coffee can speed up the metabolism. In nutritional circles, it's known as a metabolic enhancer, according to Dr. Judith Stern of the University of California at Davis.

This makes sense since caffeine is a stimulant. Studies show it can help you burn more calories than normal, perhaps up to 10 percent more. For safety's sake, it's best to limit your intake to a single cup in the morning and one in the afternoon. Add only skim milk to tit and try doing without sugar – many people learn to love it that way.

Health Benefits:

Cognitive Function:

The caffeine in coffee has been shown to enhance cognitive performance, including improved attention, memory, and reaction time. Regular coffee consumption may also reduce the risk of cognitive decline and neurodegenerative diseases such as Alzheimer's and Parkinson's disease.

Physical Performance:

Caffeine acts as an ergogenic aid, enhancing physical performance by increasing endurance, strength, and power output. It does so by stimulating the release of adrenaline and promoting the utilization of fatty acids as a fuel source during exercise.

Metabolic Health:

Coffee consumption has been associated with a reduced risk of type 2 diabetes, thanks in part to its ability to improve insulin sensitivity and glucose metabolism. The antioxidants in coffee may also play a role in protecting pancreatic beta cells from damage.

Heart Health:

Moderate coffee consumption has been linked to a lower risk of heart disease and stroke. The antioxidants in coffee help reduce inflammation, improve blood vessel function, and lower levels of LDL (bad) cholesterol.

Some studies suggest that coffee may also have a protective effect against heart rhythm disturbances and reduce the risk of heart failure.

Liver Health:

Regular coffee consumption has been associated with a reduced risk of liver diseases, including liver cirrhosis, non-alcoholic fatty liver disease (NAFLD), and liver cancer. The beneficial effects of coffee on liver health are attributed to its ability to reduce inflammation, inhibit fibrosis, and improve liver enzyme levels.

Mood and Mental Health:

Coffee is often credited with enhancing mood and promoting feelings of well-being, thanks to its ability to increase dopamine and serotonin levels in the brain. Moderate coffee consumption has been associated with a lower risk of depression and suicide.

Longevity:

Some observational studies suggest that moderate coffee consumption may be associated with a longer lifespan. The exact mechanisms underlying this association are not fully understood but may involve the antioxidant and anti-inflammatory properties of coffee.

Grapefruit

There's good reason for this traditional diet food to be a regular part of your diet. It helps dissolve fat and cholesterol, according to Dr. James Cerd of the University of Florida. An average sized grapefruit has 74 calories, delivers a whopping 15 grams of pectin (the special fiber linked to lowering cholesterol and fat), is high in vitamin C and potassium and is free of fat and sodium.

It's rich in natural galacturonic acid, which adds to its potency as a fat and cholesterol fighter. The additional benefit here is assistance in the battle against atherosclerosis (hardening of the arteries) and the development of heart disease. Try sprinkling it with cinnamon rather than sugar to take away some of the tart taste.

Nutritional Composition:

Grapefruit boasts an impressive nutritional profile, providing a rich array of vitamins, minerals, and bioactive compounds. A 100-gram serving of fresh grapefruit typically contains:

Vitamins:

Grapefruit is an excellent source of vitamin C, providing over 50% of the recommended daily intake per serving. Vitamin C plays a crucial role in immune function, collagen synthesis, and antioxidant defense.

Additionally, grapefruit contains small amounts of other vitamins, including vitamin A, vitamin B6, thiamine (vitamin B1), riboflavin (vitamin B2), and folate (vitamin B9).

Minerals:

Grapefruit contains minerals such as potassium, magnesium, calcium, and phosphorus. Potassium, in particular, helps regulate blood pressure, muscle function, and electrolyte balance.

Antioxidants:

Grapefruit is rich in antioxidants, including flavonoids, carotenoids (such as beta-carotene and lycopene), and vitamin C. These antioxidants help neutralize harmful free radicals, reduce inflammation, and protect cells from oxidative damage.

Dietary Fiber:

Grapefruit contains both soluble and insoluble fiber, which promotes digestive health, regulates bowel movements and supports weight management. Fiber also contributes to feelings of fullness and satiety, aiding in appetite control.

Health Benefits:

Immune Support:

The high vitamin C content of grapefruit makes it a potent ally in supporting immune function and combating infections, including the common cold and flu. Vitamin C stimulates the production of white blood cells and antibodies, enhancing the body's ability to fight off pathogens.

Weight Management:

Grapefruit has gained popularity as a "weight-loss" fruit due to its low calorie and high fiber content. Studies suggest that including grapefruit in meals or consuming grapefruit juice before meals may promote weight loss by reducing calorie intake, increasing feelings of fullness, and enhancing fat metabolism.

Some research indicates that compounds in grapefruit, such as naringin and hesperidin, may help regulate insulin levels and improve insulin sensitivity, which could further support weight management efforts.

Heart Health:

Regular consumption of grapefruit has been associated with a reduced risk of heart disease and stroke. The antioxidants and phytochemicals in grapefruit help lower cholesterol levels, reduce inflammation, and improve blood vessel function.

Potassium, a mineral abundant in grapefruit, helps regulate blood pressure and prevent hypertension, which is a significant risk factor for heart disease.

Digestive Health:

The fiber content in grapefruit promotes digestive health by preventing constipation, supporting regular bowel movements, and nourishing beneficial gut bacteria. Soluble fiber forms a gel-like substance in the digestive tract, which helps soften stools and ease bowel movements.

Skin Health:

The vitamin C and antioxidants in grapefruit play a vital role in maintaining healthy skin by promoting collagen synthesis, protecting against UV damage, and reducing the signs of aging such as wrinkles and fine lines. Consuming grapefruit regularly may contribute to a more youthful and radiant complexion.

Cancer Prevention:

Some studies suggest that the antioxidants and phytochemicals in grapefruit may help reduce the risk of certain types of cancer, including breast, prostate, and colon cancer. These compounds have been shown to inhibit cancer cell growth, induce apoptosis (cell death), and reduce tumor formation and metastasis.

Hydration:

With its high water content, grapefruit helps keep the body hydrated and supports optimal fluid balance. Proper hydration is essential for various physiological functions, including temperature regulation, nutrient transport, and waste elimination.

Mustard

Try the hot, spicy kind you find in Asian import stores, specialty shops, and exotic groceries. Dr. Jaya Henry of Oxford Polytechnic Institute in England found that the amount of hot mustard normally called for in Mexican, Indian, and Asian recipes, about one teaspoon, temporarily speeds up the metabolism, just as caffeine and the drug ephedrine do.

"But mustard is natural and safe," Henry says. "It can be used every day, and it works. I was shocked to discover it can speed up the metabolism by as much as 20 to 25 percent for several hours." This can result in the body burning an extra 45 calories for every 700 consumed, Dr. Henry says.

Nutritional Composition:

Mustard, derived from the seeds of the mustard plant, is a rich source of essential nutrients, including vitamins, minerals, antioxidants, and phytochemicals. A 100-gram serving of mustard seeds typically contains:

Vitamins:

Mustard seeds are abundant in vitamins, particularly vitamin A, vitamin C, vitamin K, and various B vitamins such as folate, thiamine, and riboflavin. These vitamins play essential roles in immune function, blood clotting, energy metabolism, and cellular health.

Minerals:

Mustard seeds contain minerals such as calcium, magnesium, phosphorus, potassium, and iron. These minerals are vital for bone health, muscle function, nerve transmission, and oxygen transport in the body.

Antioxidants:

Mustard seeds are rich in antioxidants, including flavonoids, phenolic compounds, and glucosinolates. These antioxidants help neutralize harmful free radicals, reduce inflammation, and protect cells from oxidative damage.

Dietary Fiber:

Mustard seeds are a good source of dietary fiber, both soluble and insoluble. Fiber promotes digestive health, regulates bowel movements, and helps control blood sugar levels. It also contributes to feelings of fullness and satiety, aiding in weight management.

Health Benefits:

Digestive Health:

The fiber content in mustard seeds supports digestive health by promoting regular bowel movements, preventing constipation, and nourishing beneficial gut bacteria. Mustard seeds also contain compounds called mucilage, which help soothe and protect the gastrointestinal tract.

Anti-inflammatory Properties:

Mustard seeds contain anti-inflammatory compounds such as selenium and magnesium, which help reduce inflammation and alleviate symptoms of inflammatory conditions such as arthritis, asthma, and inflammatory bowel disease (IBD).

Consuming mustard as part of a balanced diet may help lower levels of inflammatory markers in the body and reduce the risk of chronic inflammatory diseases.

Heart Health:

Mustard seeds are rich in omega-3 fatty acids, which have been linked to improved heart health and reduced risk of cardiovascular disease. Omega-3s help lower cholesterol levels, reduce blood pressure, and prevent blood clot formation.

Additionally, the antioxidants in mustard seeds help protect the heart from oxidative damage, reduce inflammation in the arteries, and improve blood vessel function.

Cancer Prevention:

Mustard seeds contain glucosinolates, sulfur-containing compounds that have been studied for their potential anticancer properties. Glucosinolates are converted into isothiocyanates in the body, which help inhibit cancer cell growth, induce apoptosis (cell death), and reduce tumor formation.

Some research suggests that consuming mustard regularly may help lower the risk of certain types of cancer, including colorectal, lung, and prostate cancer.

Respiratory Health:

Mustard seeds contain volatile compounds that have expectorant and decongestant properties, making them beneficial for respiratory health. Mustard seeds may help relieve symptoms of coughs, colds, bronchitis, and sinus congestion.

Inhaling the vapors of mustard seeds or mustard oil may help clear nasal passages, reduce inflammation in the respiratory tract, and improve breathing.

Skin and Hair Health:

Mustard oil, derived from mustard seeds, is rich in vitamins, minerals, and fatty acids that nourish the skin and hair. Applying mustard oil topically may help moisturize dry skin, reduce inflammation, and promote wound healing.

Mustard oil is also used in traditional Ayurvedic medicine for its antibacterial and antifungal properties, which can help treat skin infections and scalp conditions such as dandruff.

Peppers

Hot, spicy chili peppers fall into the same category as hot mustard, Henry says. He studied them under the same circumstances as the mustard and they worked just as well. A mere three grams of chili peppers were added to a meal consisting of 766 total calories. The peppers' metabolism-raising properties worked like a charm, leading to what Henry calls a diet-induced thermic effect. It doesn't take much to create the effect. Most salsa recipes call for four to eight chilies – that's not a lot.

Peppers are astonishingly rich in vitamins A and C, abundant in calcium, phosphorus, iron, and magnesium, high in fiber, free of fat, low in sodium, and have just 24 calories per cup.

Nutritional Composition of Peppers:

Peppers exhibit remarkable nutritional diversity, offering an array of essential vitamins, minerals, and phytochemicals. They are particularly rich in vitamin C, with some varieties containing more ascorbic acid than citrus fruits. This antioxidant vitamin plays a crucial role in bolstering the immune system, promoting collagen synthesis, and combating oxidative stress-induced cellular damage. Additionally, peppers are excellent sources of vitamin A, contributing to vision health, immune function, and skin integrity.

Moreover, peppers are replete with vitamin K, which is vital for blood clotting and bone metabolism, as well as vitamin B6, essential for neurotransmitter synthesis and immune modulation. They also provide notable amounts of folate, a B-vitamin crucial for DNA synthesis and red blood cell formation, making them particularly beneficial for pregnant women.

Mineral-wise, peppers contain potassium, magnesium, and manganese, all of which are integral for cardiovascular health, nerve function, and energy metabolism. Furthermore, their vibrant hues signify the presence of potent phytochemicals such as carotenoids, flavonoids, and capsaicinoids, each conferring unique health benefits.

Medicinal Properties and Health Benefits:

Antioxidant Activity:

Peppers possess potent antioxidant properties attributed to their high content of vitamin C, carotenoids, and flavonoids. These antioxidants scavenge harmful free radicals, mitigate oxidative stress, and reduce the risk of chronic diseases such as cardiovascular ailments, cancer, and neurodegenerative disorders.

Anti-inflammatory Effects:

Capsaicin, the bioactive compound responsible for the pungent heat in peppers, exhibits pronounced anti-inflammatory properties. It inhibits the activity of inflammatory mediators, alleviates pain perception, and may mitigate the symptoms of inflammatory conditions like arthritis and inflammatory bowel disease.

Cardiovascular Health:

Regular consumption of peppers has been associated with improved cardiovascular health outcomes. Their potassium content helps regulate blood pressure by counteracting the hypertensive effects of sodium, while their fiber content aids in cholesterol management and promotes satiety, thereby reducing the risk of hypertension and atherosclerosis.

Weight Management:

Peppers, particularly hot varieties containing capsaicin, have been implicated in weight management and metabolic health. Capsaicin enhances thermogenesis, increases energy expenditure, and promotes fat oxidation, potentially aiding in weight loss and adiposity reduction.

Cancer Prevention:

The diverse array of phytochemicals found in peppers exhibits promising anticancer properties. Capsaicin, in particular, has demonstrated potential in inhibiting the proliferation of cancer cells, inducing apoptosis, and suppressing tumor growth in various preclinical models. Additionally, the carotenoids and flavonoids present in peppers exert protective effects against certain cancers, including lung, prostate, and gastrointestinal malignancies.

Digestive Health:

Peppers contain dietary fiber, which supports digestive health by promoting regular bowel movements, preventing constipation, and fostering a healthy gut microbiota. Furthermore, capsaicin may stimulate gastric secretions, enhance gastrointestinal motility, and alleviate symptoms of dyspepsia and indigestion.

Vision Protection:

The high content of vitamin A and carotenoids in peppers contributes to vision health by preventing oxidative damage to the retina, reducing the risk of age-related macular degeneration, and maintaining optimal visual acuity, particularly in low-light conditions.

Immune Support:

Peppers are rich in immune-boosting nutrients such as vitamin C, which enhances the production and activity of immune cells, promotes wound healing, and protects against infections. Additionally, their antioxidant and anti-inflammatory properties fortify the immune system and mitigate the risk of chronic inflammatory diseases.

Incorporating Peppers into the Diet:

To reap the myriad health benefits offered by peppers, it is advisable to incorporate them into a balanced and varied diet. Peppers can be enjoyed raw in salads, sliced and sautéed as a side dish, stuffed with flavorful fillings, roasted for added depth of flavor, or blended into soups, sauces, and salsas. Furthermore, they can be preserved through pickling, drying, or freezing to prolong their shelf life and retain their nutritional potency.

It is important to note that individuals with sensitivities or allergies to peppers should exercise caution and consult with healthcare professionals before incorporating them into their diet. Additionally, those with gastrointestinal conditions such as GERD or irritable bowel syndrome may experience exacerbation of symptoms with spicy varieties and should consume peppers in moderation.

Potatoes

We've got to be kidding, right? Wrong. Potatoes have developed the same "fattening" rap as bread, and it's unfair. Dr. John McDougal, director of the nutritional medicine clinic at St. Helena Hospital in Deer Park, California, says, "An excellent food with which to achieve rapid weight loss is the potato, at 0.6 calories per gram or about 85 calories per potato." A great source of fiber and potassium, they lower cholesterol and protect against strokes and heart disease.

Preparation and toppings are crucial. Steer clear of butter, milk, and sour cream, or you'll blow it. Opt for yogurt instead.

Nutritional Composition of Potatoes:

Potatoes serve as a rich source of essential nutrients, including carbohydrates, vitamins, minerals, and dietary fiber. While often associated with carbohydrates, potatoes also provide protein and negligible amounts of fat, making them a valuable energy source. Notably, potatoes offer a substantial amount of vitamin C, with a single medium-sized potato fulfilling a significant portion of the daily recommended intake. Vitamin C plays a crucial role in immune function, collagen synthesis, and antioxidant defense, contributing to overall health and disease prevention.

Moreover, potatoes are abundant in potassium, a mineral essential for maintaining fluid balance, regulating blood pressure, and supporting cardiovascular health. Additionally, they contain significant amounts of vitamin B6, which is involved in amino acid metabolism, neurotransmitter synthesis, and immune modulation. Furthermore, potatoes provide folate, a B-vitamin crucial for DNA synthesis and cell division, particularly important during periods of rapid growth and development.

Potatoes also serve as a notable source of dietary fiber, with the skin containing a higher concentration than the flesh. Dietary fiber promotes digestive health, regulates bowel movements, and fosters a sense of satiety, aiding in weight management and glycemic control. Additionally, the resistant starch present in potatoes acts as a prebiotic, nourishing beneficial gut bacteria and supporting gut health.

Health Benefits of Potatoes:

Heart Health:

The potassium content of potatoes contributes to heart health by counteracting the hypertensive effects of sodium, promoting vasodilation, and regulating blood pressure. Studies have shown that diets rich in potassium are associated with a reduced risk of stroke, hypertension, and cardiovascular disease, highlighting the cardioprotective effects of potatoes.

Digestive Health:

The fiber content of potatoes supports digestive health by promoting regular bowel movements, preventing constipation, and alleviating symptoms of gastrointestinal disorders such as diverticulosis and irritable bowel syndrome. Additionally, the resistant starch in potatoes acts as a prebiotic, nourishing beneficial gut bacteria and fostering a healthy gut microbiota.

Weight Management:

Despite their reputation as a starchy vegetable, potatoes can be incorporated into a balanced diet conducive to weight management. The high fiber content of potatoes promotes satiety, reduces appetite, and curbs calorie intake, aiding in weight loss and weight maintenance efforts. Moreover, the resistant starch in potatoes may enhance feelings of fullness, regulate blood sugar levels, and increase fat oxidation, further supporting weight management goals.

Blood Sugar Regulation:

Contrary to popular belief, potatoes can be included in diabetic meal plans when consumed in appropriate portions and prepared using healthy cooking methods. The glycemic index of potatoes varies depending on factors such as cooking method and variety, with boiled or baked potatoes generally having a lower glycemic index compared to fried or processed forms. Furthermore, the fiber and resistant starch in potatoes slows down carbohydrate digestion and absorption, preventing rapid spikes in blood sugar levels and promoting glycemic control.

Skin Health:

The vitamin C content of potatoes contributes to skin health by promoting collagen synthesis, protecting against UV-induced damage, and maintaining skin elasticity and hydration. Additionally, the antioxidants present in potatoes scavenge free radicals, mitigate oxidative stress, and reduce the risk of skin aging, wrinkles, and blemishes.

Immune Support:

Potatoes are rich in immune-boosting nutrients such as vitamin C and vitamin B6, which play integral roles in immune function and defense against pathogens. By bolstering the immune system, potatoes help protect against infections, reduce the severity and duration of illness, and promote overall health and well-being.

Incorporating Potatoes into the Diet:

Potatoes can be enjoyed in a myriad of culinary preparations, ranging from simple boiled or baked dishes to more elaborate mashed, roasted, or gratin preparations. Additionally, they can be incorporated into soups, stews, salads, and casseroles, adding texture, flavor, and nutritional value to meals.

When selecting potatoes, opt for varieties with vibrant skins and firm, blemish-free flesh, as these are indicators of freshness and quality. It is advisable to store potatoes in a cool, dark, and well-ventilated place to prevent sprouting and maintain their nutritional potency.

Rice

An entire weight-loss plan, simply called the Rice Diet, was developed by Dr. William Kempner at Duke University in Durham, North Carolina. The diet, dating to the 1930s, makes rice the staple of your food intake. Later on, you gradually mix in various fruits and vegetables.

It produces stunning weight loss and medical results. The diet has been shown to reverse and cure kidney ailments and high blood pressure.

A cup of cooked rice (150 grams) contains about 178 calories – approximately one-third the number of calories found in an equivalent amount of beef or cheese. And remember, whole grain rice is much better for you than white rice.

Nutritional Composition:

Rice is a rich source of essential nutrients, including complex carbohydrates, vitamins, minerals, and dietary fiber. The specific nutritional composition varies depending on the type of rice, but in general, rice provides:

Carbohydrates:

Rice serves as a primary source of energy, supplying complex carbohydrates that fuel bodily functions and physical activity. The carbohydrates in rice are predominantly in the form of starch, which is slowly digested, providing sustained energy levels and promoting satiety.

Vitamins:

While rice is not as rich in vitamins as some other grains, it does contain small amounts of B vitamins, including thiamine (B1), riboflavin (B2), niacin (B3), and vitamin B6. These vitamins play essential roles in energy metabolism, nervous system function, and red blood cell production.

Minerals:

Rice contains several minerals, including magnesium, phosphorus, potassium, and iron. These minerals are crucial for maintaining bone health, supporting muscle function, regulating blood pressure, and preventing iron-deficiency anemia.

Dietary Fiber:

Brown rice, in particular, is a good source of dietary fiber, providing both soluble and insoluble fiber. Soluble fiber helps lower cholesterol levels and stabilize blood sugar levels, while insoluble fiber promotes digestive health and regular bowel movements.

Health Benefits:

Energy Source:

Rice serves as a primary source of energy for billions of people worldwide, providing sustained fuel for daily activities and physical exertion. Its complex carbohydrates are digested slowly, helping maintain stable blood sugar levels and preventing energy crashes.

Weight Management:

Despite its relatively high carbohydrate content, rice can be part of a healthy weight management plan when consumed in moderation and as part of a balanced diet. Its low fat and cholesterol content, combined with its high fiber content, promotes feelings of fullness and satiety, reducing overall calorie intake.

Digestive Health:

The fiber content in rice, particularly brown rice, supports digestive health by promoting regular bowel movements, preventing constipation, and reducing the risk of digestive disorders such as diverticulosis.

Additionally, the resistant starch found in cooked and cooled rice acts as a prebiotic, feeding beneficial gut bacteria and promoting a healthy microbiome.

Heart Health:

Whole grains like brown rice have been associated with a reduced risk of heart disease and stroke. The fiber, antioxidants, and phytochemicals in rice help lower cholesterol levels, reduce inflammation, and improve blood vessel function.

Studies have shown that replacing refined grains with whole grains like brown rice can lower the risk of cardiovascular disease and improve overall heart health.

Blood Sugar Control:

Brown rice, with its intact bran and germ layers, has a lower glycemic index compared to white rice, meaning it causes a slower and more gradual increase in blood sugar levels after meals. This property makes brown rice a suitable choice for individuals with diabetes or those seeking to stabilize blood sugar levels.

Nutrient Density:

Rice, especially brown rice, is a nutrient-dense food, providing essential vitamins, minerals, and antioxidants in a relatively low-calorie package. Including rice as part of a varied and balanced diet can help meet daily nutrient requirements and promote overall health and well-being.

Soups

Soup is good for you! Maybe not the canned varieties from the store – but old-fashioned, homemade soup promotes weight loss. A study by Dr. John Foreyt of Baylor College of Medicine in Houston, Texas, found that dieters who ate a bowl of soup before lunch and dinner lost more weight than dieters who didn't. The more soup they ate, the more weight they lost. And soup eaters tend to keep the weight off longer.

Naturally, the type of soup you eat makes a difference. Cream soups or those made of beef or pork are not your best bets. But here's a great recipe:

Slice three large onions, three carrots, four stalks of celery, one zucchini, and one yellow squash. Place in a kettle. Add three cans of crushed tomatoes, two packets of low-sodium chicken bouillon, three cans of water, and one cup of white wine (optional). Add tarragon, basil, oregano, thyme and garlic powder. Boil, then simmer for an hour. Serves six.

Nutritional Components of Soups:

Soups serve as a nutritional powerhouse, combining a medley of ingredients such as vegetables, legumes, grains, meats, and herbs into a nourishing and flavorful concoction. The nutritional composition of soups varies widely depending on the ingredients used, but they often encompass a balance of macronutrients, vitamins, minerals, and phytochemicals essential for optimal health.

Macronutrients:

Soups typically contain a blend of carbohydrates, proteins, and fats, providing a source of sustained energy and satiety. Carbohydrates from ingredients such as vegetables, grains, and legumes serve as the primary energy source, while proteins from meats, legumes, and dairy products contribute to muscle repair and growth. Healthy fats, derived from sources like olive oil or avocado, offer essential fatty acids crucial for cell membrane integrity, hormone synthesis, and nutrient absorption.

Vitamins and Minerals:

Vegetable-based soups are rich in vitamins and minerals, particularly vitamins A, C, and K, as well as potassium, magnesium, and folate. These micronutrients play integral roles in immune function, bone health, cardiovascular health, and overall vitality. Additionally, the slow simmering process of soups helps release nutrients from ingredients, enhancing their bioavailability and facilitating absorption by the body.

Phytochemicals:

Soups abound with phytochemicals and bioactive compounds found in plant-based foods that confer numerous health benefits. Ingredients such as tomatoes, garlic, onions, leafy greens, and herbs are replete with antioxidants, anti-inflammatory agents, and immune-modulating compounds that help protect against chronic diseases, bolster immune function, and promote longevity.

Health Benefits of Soups:

Hydration and Fluid Balance:

Soups, being primarily water-based, contribute to hydration and fluid balance, especially important for maintaining optimal physiological function and supporting cellular processes. Consuming soups can help prevent dehydration, particularly in individuals who struggle to meet their daily fluid intake requirements.

Digestive Health:

The liquid consistency of soups, combined with the high fiber content of vegetable-based varieties, supports digestive health by promoting regular bowel movements, preventing constipation, and fostering a healthy gut microbiota. Additionally, the warm temperature of soups can soothe the digestive tract and alleviate symptoms of gastrointestinal discomfort.

Weight Management:

Incorporating soups into a balanced diet can aid in weight management and appetite control. The high water content and fiber-rich ingredients of soups promote satiety, reduce hunger cues, and lower overall calorie intake. Moreover, soups can be a nutrient-dense and low-energy-density option, allowing individuals to satisfy their appetites while consuming fewer calories.

Immune Support:

Soups brimming with nutrient-rich ingredients such as vegetables, herbs, and lean proteins provide essential nutrients and phytochemicals that bolster immune function and enhance resilience against infections. The vitamins, minerals, and antioxidants present in soups play integral roles in immune modulation, inflammation regulation, and pathogen defense.

Heart Health:

Homemade soups prepared with wholesome ingredients and minimal added sodium can contribute to heart health by promoting blood pressure regulation, cholesterol management, and overall cardiovascular function. Ingredients like beans, lentils, whole grains, and vegetables are rich in fiber, potassium, and heart-healthy fats, which help lower cholesterol levels, reduce inflammation, and support vascular health.

Bone Health:

Soups enriched with bone broth or fortified with calcium-rich ingredients like leafy greens and dairy products can support bone health and prevent osteoporosis. The minerals and collagen peptides present in bone broth contribute to bone strength, density, and resilience, while calcium and vitamin D aid in calcium absorption and bone mineralization.

Mental Well-being:

Beyond their physical health benefits, soups nourish the soul and uplift the spirit, offering comfort, warmth, and a sense of culinary satisfaction. The act of preparing and sharing soups fosters social connections, promotes mindfulness, and provides a source of emotional nourishment during times of stress or uncertainty.

Incorporating Soups into the Diet:

Soups offer endless culinary possibilities and can be customized to suit individual tastes, dietary preferences, and nutritional goals. Whether enjoyed as a light starter, hearty main course, or wholesome snack, soups can be adapted to accommodate various dietary restrictions, cultural traditions, and seasonal ingredients.

To maximize the nutritional benefits of soups, opt for homemade varieties prepared with fresh, whole ingredients and minimal added sodium, preservatives, or artificial additives. Experiment with different flavor profiles, textures, and cooking techniques to create soups that delight the palate and nourish the body.

Spinach

Popeye knew what he was talking about, according to Dr. Richard Shekelle, an epidemiologist at the University of Texas. Spinach can lower cholesterol, rev up the metabolism, and burn away fat. Rich in iron, beta-carotene, and vitamins C and E, it supplies most of the nutrients you need.

Nutritional Composition:

Spinach is renowned for its rich and diverse nutritional profile, boasting an impressive array of vitamins, minerals, antioxidants, and other bioactive compounds. A 100-gram serving of raw spinach typically contains:

Vitamins:

Spinach is a potent source of vitamins, particularly vitamin A (in the form of beta-carotene), vitamin K, vitamin C, and folate (vitamin B9). These vitamins play essential roles in various bodily functions, including vision, immune function, blood clotting, and DNA synthesis.

Minerals:

Spinach is rich in minerals such as iron, calcium, magnesium, potassium, and manganese. These minerals are critical for maintaining bone health, muscle function, electrolyte balance, and overall metabolic processes.

Antioxidants:

Spinach contains a variety of antioxidants, including flavonoids, carotenoids (such as lutein and zeaxanthin), and phenolic compounds. These antioxidants help neutralize harmful free radicals, reduce inflammation, and protect cells from oxidative damage.

Dietary Fiber:

Spinach is an excellent source of dietary fiber, both soluble and insoluble, which promotes digestive health, regulates bowel movements, and helps control blood sugar levels. Fiber also contributes to feelings of fullness and satiety, aiding in weight management.

Health Benefits:

Heart Health:

The abundance of vitamins, minerals, and antioxidants in spinach contributes to heart health by reducing inflammation, lowering blood pressure, and preventing oxidative stress. The high levels of potassium and magnesium in spinach help regulate blood pressure and promote healthy cardiovascular function.

Bone Health:

Spinach is rich in vitamin K, which is essential for bone health and calcium metabolism. Vitamin K plays a crucial role in bone mineralization and helps prevent osteoporosis and fractures.

Additionally, the calcium and magnesium content of spinach contribute to bone strength and density, further supporting skeletal health.

Eye Health:

Lutein and zeaxanthin, two carotenoids found abundantly in spinach, are known to promote eye health by protecting against age-related macular degeneration (AMD) and cataracts. These antioxidants help filter harmful blue light and reduce oxidative damage to the eyes.

Cancer Prevention:

Spinach contains various phytochemicals with anticancer properties, including flavonoids, carotenoids, and chlorophyll. These compounds help inhibit the growth of cancer cells, induce apoptosis (cell death), and reduce tumor formation and metastasis.

Regular consumption of spinach has been associated with a reduced risk of several types of cancer, including breast, prostate, colorectal, and lung cancer.

Blood Sugar Control:

The fiber and antioxidants in spinach help regulate blood sugar levels and improve insulin sensitivity, making it beneficial for individuals with diabetes or those at risk of developing the condition. Spinach has a low glycemic index, meaning it causes a gradual rise in blood sugar levels after consumption.

Weight Management:

Spinach is low in calories and carbohydrates but high in fiber and water content, making it an ideal food for weight management. The fiber and water in spinach add bulk to meals, promoting feelings of fullness and reducing overall calorie intake.

Including spinach in meals and snacks can help control appetite, prevent overeating, and support weight loss or maintenance goals.

Tofu

You just can't say enough about this healthy food from Asia. Also called soybean curd, it's tasteless, so any spice or flavoring you add blends with it nicely. A 2½ " square has 86 calories and nine grams of protein. (Experts suggest an intake of about 40 grams per day.) Tofu contains calcium and iron, almost no sodium, and not a bit of saturated fat. It makes your metabolism run on high and even lowers cholesterol. With different varieties available, the firmer tofus are good for stir-frying or adding to soups and sauces while the softer ones are good for mashing, chopping, and adding to salads.

Nutritional Profile of Tofu:

Tofu is a nutrient-dense food, packed with essential vitamins, minerals, and macronutrients. It serves as an excellent source of plant-based protein, offering all nine essential amino acids required for human health. Moreover, tofu is low in saturated fat and cholesterol-free, making it a heart-healthy alternative to animal-based protein sources. Additionally, tofu contains significant amounts of calcium, iron, magnesium, phosphorus, and other essential minerals crucial for maintaining bone health, muscle function, and overall vitality.

Protein Powerhouse:

One of the most significant benefits of tofu is its high protein content. Protein is essential for building and repairing tissues, supporting immune function, and maintaining healthy skin, hair, and nails. Tofu provides approximately 8 grams of protein per 100-gram serving, making it an excellent protein source for vegetarians, vegans, and individuals looking to reduce their meat consumption. The protein in tofu is also easily digestible and can contribute to satiety, helping to control appetite and promote weight management.

Heart Health:

Consuming tofu regularly may have positive effects on heart health. Tofu is rich in polyunsaturated fats, particularly omega-3 fatty acids, which have been linked to reduced risk factors for cardiovascular disease, such as lower levels of LDL cholesterol and triglycerides. Moreover, the absence of cholesterol in tofu makes it a heart-healthy alternative to animal-based protein sources, which can contribute to elevated cholesterol levels and increased risk of heart disease. Including tofu in a balanced diet may help lower blood pressure, improve blood lipid profiles, and reduce the risk of heart attacks and strokes.

Bone Health:

Tofu contains high levels of calcium and other minerals essential for bone health. Adequate calcium intake is crucial for maintaining strong and healthy bones, reducing the risk of osteoporosis and fractures, especially as individuals age. Tofu made with calcium sulfate provides a significant amount of bioavailable calcium, making it an excellent dietary source for individuals who cannot consume dairy products or prefer plant-based alternatives. Additionally, the presence of magnesium, phosphorus, and vitamin D in tofu further supports bone mineralization and overall skeletal integrity.

Cancer Prevention:

Emerging research suggests that incorporating tofu into your diet may help reduce the risk of certain types of cancer. Soybeans contain phytochemicals called isoflavones, which exhibit antioxidant and anti-cancer properties. Genistein, daidzein, and other isoflavones found in tofu have been studied for their potential role in inhibiting cancer cell growth, particularly breast, prostate, and colorectal cancers. While more research is needed to fully understand the mechanisms behind soy's anti-cancer effects, observational studies have shown promising associations between soy consumption and reduced cancer incidence in populations with high tofu intake.

Hormonal Balance:

Contrary to some misconceptions, moderate consumption of tofu does not appear to have adverse effects on hormonal balance or reproductive health. Soy isoflavones, particularly genistein and daidzein, have been studied for their phytoestrogenic properties, which can mimic or modulate the effects of estrogen in the body. While concerns have been raised about potential estrogenic effects interfering with hormone levels, clinical trials, and meta-analyses have generally found that moderate soy consumption is safe and may even offer protective effects against hormone-related conditions such as breast cancer, menopausal symptoms, and osteoporosis.

Weight Management:

Incorporating tofu into a balanced diet may support weight management and healthy body composition. Tofu is low in calories and saturated fat while being high in protein and fiber, both of which contribute to increased satiety and reduced calorie intake. Including tofu in meals can help prevent overeating, promote feelings of fullness, and support weight loss or weight maintenance goals. Additionally, the versatility of tofu allows for a wide range of culinary applications, making it easy to incorporate into various dishes as a nutritious and satisfying ingredient.

Diabetes Management:

Tofu may offer benefits for individuals with diabetes or those at risk of developing the condition. The low glycemic index of tofu means it has minimal impact on blood sugar levels, making it suitable for inclusion in diabetic-friendly meal plans. Furthermore, the protein and fiber content of tofu can help stabilize blood glucose levels, improve insulin sensitivity, and reduce the risk of insulin resistance and type 2 diabetes. By replacing high-carbohydrate foods with tofu-based alternatives, individuals with diabetes can better manage their blood sugar levels and overall health.

Digestive Health:

Tofu contains dietary fiber, which plays a crucial role in supporting digestive health and preventing constipation. Fiber adds bulk to stool, promotes regular bowel movements, and nourishes beneficial gut bacteria, thereby maintaining a healthy gastrointestinal tract. Additionally, the probiotics and prebiotics found in fermented tofu products such as tempeh contribute to gut microbiome diversity and function, further enhancing digestive wellness. Including tofu and other soy-based foods in your diet can help promote optimal digestion and overall gastrointestinal comfort.

Potent Foods

It would be unrealistic to think you could successfully lose weight and enjoy what you're eating with a mere handful of foods, no matter how delicious, nutritious, and satisfying they may be. So we're going to add an extra roster of fat-fighting foods you can eat along with the great foods mentioned in the last section.

They'll lend different tastes and textures to every meal and provide a wide range of vitamins, minerals, proteins, and other vital nutrients. Naturally, each one is high in fiber, low in fat, and safe when it comes to sodium content, too.

Many have the crunchiness and flavor we've come to desire in snack and nibbling foods. If you're like most of us, you may have a real junk food snacking habit – a habit you're going to have to change to slim down. Many of the foods in this section may be worthy substitutes.

Barley

This filling grain stacks up favorably with rice and potatoes. It has 170 calories per cooked cup, respectable levels of protein and fiber, and relatively low fat. Roman gladiators ate this grain regularly for strength and complained when they had to eat meat.

Studies at the University of Wisconsin show that barley effectively lowers cholesterol by up to 15 percent and has powerful anti-cancer agents. Israeli scientists say it cures constipation better than laxatives - and that can promote weight loss, too.

Nutrient Composition:

Barley boasts an impressive nutritional profile, rich in essential vitamins, minerals, fiber, and antioxidants. A 100-gram serving of cooked barley provides approximately 193 calories, consisting mainly of complex carbohydrates, along with moderate amounts of protein and minimal fat content. Furthermore, barley serves as an excellent source of dietary fiber, particularly beta-glucan, a soluble fiber known for its cholesterol-lowering properties. Additionally, barley contains essential micronutrients such as manganese, selenium, phosphorus, copper, and vitamins B1 (thiamine) and B3 (niacin), contributing to overall health and vitality.

Heart Health:

One of the most notable benefits of barley is its ability to promote heart health. The soluble fiber present in barley, primarily beta-glucan, helps reduce LDL (bad) cholesterol levels by interfering with its absorption in the intestines. By lowering LDL cholesterol, barley contributes to a decreased risk of cardiovascular diseases such as heart attacks and strokes. Moreover, barley contains antioxidants such as vitamin E and selenium, which combat oxidative stress and inflammation, further supporting cardiovascular health.

Blood Sugar Management:

Barley offers significant advantages for individuals managing blood sugar levels, particularly those with diabetes or insulin resistance. The soluble fiber in barley slows down the digestion and absorption of carbohydrates, leading to a gradual release of glucose into the bloodstream. This helps prevent spikes in blood sugar levels after meals, promoting better glycemic control. Studies have demonstrated that incorporating barley into the diet can improve insulin sensitivity and reduce the risk of type 2 diabetes.

Weight Management:

Incorporating barley into a balanced diet can be beneficial for weight management and satiety. The high fiber content of barley helps promote feelings of fullness and reduces hunger, which can aid in controlling calorie intake and preventing overeating. Furthermore, barley has a low glycemic index (GI), meaning it does not cause rapid fluctuations in blood sugar levels. By providing sustained energy and promoting satiety, barley can support weight loss efforts and help individuals maintain a healthy body weight.

Digestive Health:

Barley's abundant fiber content plays a crucial role in maintaining digestive health and preventing common gastrointestinal issues. The insoluble fiber in barley adds bulk to stool, promoting regularity and alleviating constipation. Additionally, the soluble fiber in barley serves as a prebiotic, nourishing beneficial gut bacteria and promoting a healthy gut microbiome. A healthy gut microbiome is associated with improved digestion, enhanced nutrient absorption, and a reduced risk of digestive disorders such as irritable bowel syndrome (IBS) and diverticulitis.

Cancer Prevention:

Emerging research suggests that barley may possess potential anticancer properties, thanks to its rich antioxidant content and other bioactive compounds. Antioxidants such as selenium, vitamin E, and phenolic acids help neutralize free radicals and inhibit oxidative damage to cells, which is implicated in the development of cancer. Furthermore, barley contains phytonutrients like lignans, which have been studied for their potential anti-cancer effects, particularly in hormone-related cancers such as breast and prostate cancer. While more research is needed to fully elucidate barley's role in cancer prevention, preliminary studies show promising results.

Bone Health:

Maintaining strong and healthy bones is essential for overall well-being, especially as we age. Barley contains several nutrients that contribute to bone health, including calcium, magnesium, phosphorus, and vitamin K. These nutrients play key roles in bone formation, mineralization, and maintenance of bone density. Additionally, the presence of silicon in barley may further enhance bone health by promoting collagen synthesis and bone mineralization. Including barley in the diet as part of a bone-friendly eating pattern can help reduce the risk of osteoporosis and fractures.

Antioxidant Properties:

Barley is a rich source of antioxidants, which are compounds that help protect cells from damage caused by free radicals and oxidative stress. The antioxidants found in barley, including vitamin E, selenium, phenolic acids, and flavonoids, exhibit potent scavenging activity against free radicals, reducing the risk of chronic diseases and premature aging. Regular consumption of antioxidant-rich foods like barley can bolster the body's defense mechanisms and support overall health and longevity.

Versatile Culinary Uses:

Beyond its nutritional benefits, barley's versatility in the kitchen makes it a valuable ingredient in various culinary preparations. From hearty soups and stews to flavorful salads and pilafs, barley lends itself well to a wide range of dishes. Its chewy texture and nutty flavor add depth and complexity to both savory and sweet recipes. Barley can also be ground into flour for baking bread, muffins, and other baked goods, offering a wholesome alternative to refined grains. With its culinary versatility and nutritional prowess, barley deserves a place of honor in any well-rounded diet.

Use it as a substitute for rice in salads, pilaf, or stuffing, or add to soups and stews. You can also mix it with rice for an interesting texture. Ground into flour, it makes excellent breads and muffins.

Beans

Beans are one of the best sources of plant protein. Peas, beans, and chickpeas are collectively known as legumes. Most common beans have 215 calories per cooked cup (lima beans go up to 260). They have the most protein with the least fat of any food, and they're high in potassium but low in sodium.

Plant protein is incomplete, which means that you need to add something to make it complete. Combine beans with whole grains – rice, barley, wheat, corn – to provide the amino acids necessary to form a complete protein. Then you get the same top-quality protein as in meat with just a fraction of the fat.

Studies at the University of Kentucky and in the Netherlands show that eating beans regularly can lower cholesterol levels.

The most common complaint about beans is that they cause gas. Here's how to contain that problem, according to the U.S. Department of Agriculture (USDA): Before cooking, rinse the beans and remove foreign particles, put in a kettle and cover with boiling water, soak for four hours or longer, remove any beans that float to the top, then cook the beans in fresh water.

Nutritional Composition of Beans:

Beans are nutritional powerhouses, rich in essential nutrients that contribute to optimal health. Here's a breakdown of their nutritional composition:

1.1 Protein:

Beans are an excellent source of plant-based protein, making them an essential component of vegetarian and vegan diets.

They contain all nine essential amino acids, although in varying proportions, making them complementary to grains for achieving complete protein intake.

Protein content varies among different types of beans, with some varieties like soybeans boasting exceptionally high protein levels.

1.2 Fiber:

Beans are renowned for their high fiber content, which promotes digestive health and helps regulate blood sugar levels.

Both soluble and insoluble fiber are present in beans, contributing to satiety, aiding in weight management, and reducing the risk of chronic diseases such as heart disease and diabetes.

1.3 Vitamins and Minerals:

Beans are rich sources of various vitamins and minerals, including folate, potassium, magnesium, iron, and zinc.

Folate is particularly abundant in beans and is crucial for cell division and DNA synthesis, making it vital for pregnant women to support fetal development.

1.4 Antioxidants:

Beans contain a diverse array of antioxidants, including flavonoids, phenolic compounds, and carotenoids, which help neutralize harmful free radicals and reduce inflammation.

Antioxidants in beans have been linked to a lower risk of chronic diseases such as cancer, cardiovascular disease, and neurodegenerative disorders.

Health Benefits of Beans:

The consumption of beans offers a wide range of health benefits, contributing to overall well-being and disease prevention. Let's explore some of the notable advantages:

2.1 Heart Health:

The high fiber content in beans helps lower cholesterol levels by binding to cholesterol and promoting its excretion.

Beans are low in saturated fat and cholesterol, making them heart-healthy alternatives to animal-based proteins.

Potassium and magnesium in beans support cardiovascular health by regulating blood pressure and promoting vasodilation.

2.2 Weight Management:

The combination of protein and fiber in beans promotes feelings of fullness and satiety, reducing overall calorie intake and aiding in weight management.

Beans have a low glycemic index, meaning they cause a gradual rise in blood sugar levels, preventing spikes and crashes that can contribute to overeating.

2.3 Diabetes Management:

The soluble fiber in beans slows down the absorption of glucose, helping stabilize blood sugar levels and reducing the risk of insulin resistance.

Beans have been associated with improved glycemic control and reduced risk of type 2 diabetes when incorporated into a balanced diet.

2.4 Digestive Health:

The high fiber content in beans promotes regular bowel movements, prevents constipation, and supports a healthy gut microbiota.

Resistant starches present in beans act as prebiotics, nourishing beneficial gut bacteria and promoting digestive health.

2.5 Cancer Prevention:

The antioxidants and phytochemicals found in beans possess anti-carcinogenic properties, helping protect against various types of cancer, including colon, breast, and prostate cancer.

Fiber in beans binds to potential carcinogens and toxins in the colon, reducing their exposure to the intestinal lining and lowering cancer risk.

Culinary Versatility of Beans:

One of the most appealing aspects of beans is their versatility in the kitchen. From soups and stews to salads and dips, beans can be incorporated into a wide range of dishes, adding flavor, texture, and nutritional value. Here are some popular ways to enjoy beans:

3.1 Soups and Stews:

Beans add heartiness and protein to soups and stews, such as minestrone, chili, and lentil soup.

They can be cooked from dried or used canned for convenience, making them ideal for quick and nutritious meals.

3.2 Salads:

Beans lend texture and protein to salads, whether tossed with leafy greens, vegetables, and vinaigrette or mixed with grains like quinoa or bulgur.

Bean salads are versatile and can be served cold or at room temperature, making them perfect for picnics and potlucks.

3.3 Dips and Spreads:

Beans can be pureed into creamy dips and spreads, such as hummus (made from chickpeas), black bean dip, or white bean spread.

These nutritious dips are excellent for snacking, spreading on sandwiches, or serving as appetizers at parties.

3.4 Main Dishes:

Beans can take center stage in vegetarian and vegan main dishes, such as bean burgers, bean-based curries, and bean casseroles.

They can be seasoned and spiced in various ways to create flavorful and satisfying meals for individuals of all dietary preferences.

Berries

This is the perfect weight-loss food. Berries have natural fructose sugar that satisfies your longing for sweets and enough fiber so you absorb fewer calories that you eat. British researchers found that the high content of insoluble fiber in fruits, vegetables, and whole grains reduces the absorption of calories from foods enough to promote width loss without hampering nutrition.

Berries are a great source of potassium that can assist you in blood pressure control. Blackberries have 74 calories per cup, blueberries 81, raspberries 60, and strawberries 45. So use your imagination and enjoy the berry of your choice.

Nutritional Profile of Berries:

Berries are low in calories and high in fiber, making them an excellent choice for weight management and digestive health.

They are rich in essential vitamins such as vitamin C, vitamin K, and various B vitamins, which play crucial roles in immune function, blood clotting, and energy metabolism.

Berries are also abundant sources of minerals like manganese, which supports bone health and antioxidant defense systems.

Antioxidant Powerhouse:

One of the most remarkable features of berries is their high antioxidant content. Antioxidants are compounds that help neutralize harmful free radicals in the body, thus reducing oxidative stress and inflammation.

Anthocyanins, flavonoids, and phenolic acids are some of the key antioxidants found in berries, contributing to their vibrant colors and health-promoting properties.

Research suggests that regular consumption of berries may help protect against chronic diseases such as heart disease, cancer, and neurodegenerative disorders by combating oxidative damage and inflammation.

Heart Health Benefits:

Berries have been linked to improvements in cardiovascular health, primarily due to their ability to lower risk factors such as high blood pressure, cholesterol levels, and inflammation.

Studies have shown that diets rich in berries are associated with a reduced risk of heart attacks, strokes, and other cardiovascular events.

The presence of flavonoids and other bioactive compounds in berries may help improve blood vessel function, promote healthy circulation, and protect against atherosclerosis.

Brain Boosting Properties:

Emerging research suggests that regular consumption of berries may have cognitive benefits, including enhanced memory, attention, and cognitive function.

Anthocyanins and other antioxidants found in berries have been shown to protect brain cells from oxidative stress and inflammation, potentially reducing the risk of age-related cognitive decline and neurodegenerative diseases like Alzheimer's.

Incorporating berries into the diet, either fresh, frozen, or dried, may offer neuroprotective effects and support overall brain health throughout life.

Diabetes Management:

Despite their natural sweetness, berries have a relatively low glycemic index, meaning they have minimal impact on blood sugar levels when consumed in moderation.

The fiber content in berries helps slow down the absorption of sugar into the bloodstream, promoting better blood sugar control and insulin sensitivity.

Some studies suggest that regular consumption of berries may reduce the risk of type 2 diabetes and its complications by improving glucose metabolism and reducing insulin resistance.

Anti-Inflammatory Effects:

Chronic inflammation is a common underlying factor in many chronic diseases, including arthritis, obesity, and heart disease. Berries possess anti-inflammatory properties that may help mitigate inflammation and its associated health risks.

Anthocyanins and other bioactive compounds in berries have been shown to inhibit inflammatory pathways in the body, thereby reducing the production of pro-inflammatory molecules.

Including a variety of berries in the diet may help modulate the body's inflammatory response and promote overall health and well-being.

Digestive Health Promotion:

The high fiber content in berries supports digestive health by promoting regular bowel movements, preventing constipation, and supporting healthy gut microbiota.

Berries contain both soluble and insoluble fiber, which contribute to feelings of fullness, regulate blood sugar levels, and nourish beneficial gut bacteria.

Regular consumption of berries may reduce the risk of digestive disorders such as diverticulitis, inflammatory bowel disease, and colorectal cancer.

Skin Health and Anti-Aging Benefits:

The antioxidant-rich nature of berries extends to their potential benefits for skin health and beauty. Antioxidants help protect skin cells from damage caused by environmental stressors such as UV radiation and pollution.

Vitamins like vitamin C found in berries play a crucial role in collagen synthesis, which is essential for maintaining skin elasticity and preventing premature aging.

Incorporating berries into the diet may promote a youthful complexion, reduce the appearance of wrinkles and age spots, and support overall skin health from within.

Cancer Prevention and Supportive Therapy:

Several studies have investigated the potential role of berries in cancer prevention and treatment. The antioxidant and anti-inflammatory properties of berries may help inhibit tumor growth and reduce cancer risk.

Compounds like ellagic acid, found in raspberries and strawberries, have been shown to exert anti-cancer effects by inducing apoptosis (programmed cell death) in cancer cells and inhibiting angiogenesis (the formation of new blood vessels that supply tumors).

While berries alone cannot cure cancer, they may complement conventional cancer treatments and support overall health during cancer treatment and recovery.

Practical Tips for Enjoying Berries:

Incorporate a variety of berries into your diet for maximum nutritional benefits. Enjoy them fresh, frozen, or dried, and include them in smoothies, salads, yogurt, oatmeal, and desserts.

Choose organic berries whenever possible to minimize exposure to pesticides and maximize nutrient content.

Experiment with different berry combinations to discover new flavors and textures. Mix and match strawberries, blueberries, raspberries, blackberries, and other varieties to create delicious and nutritious meals and snacks.

Consider growing your berries at home if space and climate permit. Homegrown berries are often fresher, tastier, and more affordable than store-bought options.

Be mindful of portion sizes, as even healthy foods like berries can contribute to calorie intake if consumed excessively. Aim for a balanced diet that includes a variety of fruits, vegetables, whole grains, lean proteins, and healthy fats.

Broccoli

Broccoli is America's favorite vegetable, according to a recent poll. No wonder. A cup of cooked broccoli has a mere 44 calories. It delivers a staggering nutritional payload and is considered the number one cancer-fighting vegetable. It has no fat, loads of fiber, cancer-fighting chemicals called indoles, and carotene, and 21 times the RDA of vitamin C and calcium.

When you're buying broccoli, pay attention to the color. The tiny florets should be rich green and free of yellowing. Stems should be firm.

Nutritional Profile:

Broccoli belongs to the cruciferous vegetable family, renowned for its exceptional nutritional density. A single cup of chopped broccoli (approximately 91 grams) contains a mere 31 calories, making it a guilt-free addition to any diet. Despite its low-calorie content, broccoli is brimming with essential nutrients, including:

Vitamin C: A potent antioxidant vital for immune function and collagen synthesis.

Vitamin K: Essential for blood clotting and bone health.

Folate: Crucial for DNA synthesis and cell division.

Fiber: Promotes digestive health and aids in weight management.

Potassium: Supports heart health and regulates blood pressure.

Calcium: Contributes to bone strength and muscle function.

Iron: Facilitates oxygen transport and energy production within cells.

Cancer Prevention Properties:

One of the most extensively studied health benefits of broccoli is its potential to reduce the risk of various types of cancer. Sulforaphane, a sulfur-containing compound abundant in broccoli, has garnered significant attention for its potent anti-cancer properties. Research suggests that sulforaphane may:

Inhibit the proliferation of cancer cells.

Induce apoptosis (programmed cell death) in malignant cells.

Detoxify carcinogenic substances and enhance their excretion from the body.

Suppress the formation of tumors in animal models.

Reduce inflammation, which is closely linked to cancer development.

Heart Health Promotion:

Consuming broccoli regularly may confer protective effects against cardiovascular diseases, the leading cause of mortality worldwide. The fiber, antioxidants, and anti-inflammatory compounds present in broccoli contribute to heart health by:

Lowering levels of LDL cholesterol, or "bad" cholesterol, thus reducing the risk of atherosclerosis.

Improving endothelial function and promoting vasodilation, helps maintain healthy blood pressure levels.

Modulating inflammatory pathways and reducing oxidative stress, both of which are implicated in the development of cardiovascular diseases.

Digestive Health Benefits:

Broccoli contains a significant amount of dietary fiber, which plays a pivotal role in maintaining digestive health and preventing constipation. Fiber adds bulk to stool, facilitating its passage through the gastrointestinal tract and promoting regular bowel movements. Additionally, broccoli contains glucosinolates, sulfur-containing compounds that support the growth of beneficial gut bacteria. A healthy gut microbiota is essential for nutrient absorption, immune function, and overall well-being.

Vision Support:

The high content of vitamin A and lutein in broccoli makes it particularly beneficial for eye health. Vitamin A is essential for maintaining optimal vision, particularly in low-light conditions, while lutein protects the eyes from oxidative damage caused by exposure to harmful ultraviolet (UV) radiation and blue light. Regular consumption of broccoli may help reduce the risk of age-related macular degeneration (AMD) and cataracts, two prevalent eye disorders associated with aging.

Anti-inflammatory Properties:

Chronic inflammation is implicated in the pathogenesis of numerous diseases, including arthritis, diabetes, and cardiovascular disorders. Broccoli contains various compounds, such as sulforaphane, quercetin, and kaempferol, that possess potent anti-inflammatory properties. These compounds inhibit the activity of pro-inflammatory enzymes and cytokines, thereby attenuating the inflammatory response and mitigating tissue damage.

Weight Management Support:

For individuals striving to achieve or maintain a healthy weight, broccoli is an excellent dietary choice. Its low-calorie and high-fiber content promotes satiety, helping curb hunger and reduce calorie intake. Furthermore, broccoli is rich in water, which adds volume to meals without contributing significant calories. Incorporating broccoli into a balanced diet can aid in weight management by promoting feelings of fullness and preventing overeating.

Bone Health Enhancement:

Maintaining strong and healthy bones is essential for overall mobility and quality of life, especially as we age. Broccoli contains a potent combination of calcium, vitamin K, and other micronutrients crucial for bone health. Calcium provides the structural framework for bones, while vitamin K regulates calcium metabolism and supports bone mineralization. Regular consumption of broccoli may help reduce the risk of osteoporosis and fractures, particularly in postmenopausal women at higher risk of bone loss.

Buckwheat

It's great for pancakes, bread, cereal, soups, or alone as a grain dish commonly called kasha. It has 155 calories per cooked cup. Research at the All India Institute of Medical Sciences shows diets including buckwheat lead to excellent blood sugar regulation, resistance to diabetes, and lowered cholesterol levels. You cook buckwheat the same way you would rice or barley. Bring two to three cups of water to a boil, add the grain, cover the pan, turn down the heat, and simmer for 20 minutes or until the water is absorbed.

Nutritional Profile:

Buckwheat is celebrated for its exceptional nutritional density, offering a wide array of essential vitamins, minerals, antioxidants, and dietary fiber. A single cup (about 168 grams) of cooked buckwheat groats provides:

Protein: Buckwheat is a notable source of plant-based protein, containing all nine essential amino acids, making it a valuable addition to vegetarian and vegan diets.

Fiber: Rich in both soluble and insoluble fiber, buckwheat supports digestive health, regulates blood sugar levels, and promotes satiety, aiding in weight management.

Complex Carbohydrates: Buckwheat's complex carbohydrates provide sustained energy release, making it an ideal choice for maintaining stable blood glucose levels.

Vitamins and Minerals: Buckwheat is a good source of magnesium, iron, zinc, manganese, phosphorus, and B-complex vitamins, including niacin, folate, and pyridoxine (vitamin B6).

Heart Health Promotion:

Regular consumption of buckwheat has been associated with numerous benefits for cardiovascular health. Several components of buckwheat, including fiber, magnesium, and antioxidants such as rutin and quercetin, contribute to heart health by:

Lowering LDL cholesterol levels and improving the ratio of HDL to LDL cholesterol, thus reducing the risk of atherosclerosis and coronary artery disease.

Regulating blood pressure levels through vasodilation and inhibition of angiotensin-converting enzyme (ACE), a key enzyme involved in blood pressure regulation.

Protecting against oxidative stress and inflammation, both of which are implicated in the development and progression of cardiovascular diseases.

Blood Sugar Regulation:

Buckwheat is renowned for its ability to help manage blood sugar levels, making it a valuable dietary choice for individuals with diabetes or those at risk of developing the condition. The combination of soluble fiber, magnesium, and polyphenolic compounds in buckwheat exerts beneficial effects on blood glucose control by:

Slowing down the absorption of carbohydrates and reducing the postprandial glycemic response, helps prevent spikes in blood sugar levels.

Improving insulin sensitivity and enhancing glucose uptake by peripheral tissues, thereby reducing insulin resistance and promoting glycemic control.

Supporting pancreatic function and insulin secretion, is crucial for maintaining glucose homeostasis.

Digestive Health Benefits:

Buckwheat's high fiber content and unique composition of phytonutrients contribute to digestive health and alleviate common gastrointestinal issues. The insoluble fiber in buckwheat promotes regular bowel movements, prevents constipation, and supports overall digestive function. Additionally, buckwheat contains resistant starch, a type of carbohydrate that acts as a prebiotic, nourishing beneficial gut bacteria and promoting a healthy gut microbiome.

Antioxidant Properties:

Buckwheat is rich in antioxidants, including flavonoids such as rutin, quercetin, and kaempferol, which possess potent free radical-scavenging activity. These antioxidants help protect cells from oxidative damage caused by reactive oxygen species (ROS), thereby reducing the risk of chronic diseases, including cancer, cardiovascular disorders, and neurodegenerative conditions. Rutin, in particular, is renowned for its anti-inflammatory and vasoprotective effects, making buckwheat a valuable dietary addition for individuals seeking to enhance their antioxidant defenses.

Gluten-Free Alternative:

For individuals with gluten intolerance or celiac disease, buckwheat serves as an excellent gluten-free alternative to wheat and other gluten-containing grains. Buckwheat is naturally gluten-free and can be incorporated into various recipes, including bread, pancakes, noodles, and baked goods, providing a nutritious and flavorful option for those following a gluten-free diet.

Weight Management Support:

Due to its high protein and fiber content, buckwheat promotes satiety and helps control appetite, making it a valuable ally in weight management efforts. Including buckwheat in meals can help reduce calorie intake, prevent overeating, and support long-term weight loss goals. Additionally, buckwheat's low glycemic index (GI) and slow digestion rate contribute to stable blood sugar levels, further aiding in weight management and metabolic health.

Versatile Culinary Uses:

Buckwheat's versatility extends beyond its nutritional benefits, as it can be incorporated into a wide range of dishes, both savory and sweet. From hearty soups and salads to nourishing porridges and desserts, buckwheat adds texture, flavor, and nutritional value to culinary creations. Buckwheat flour, groats, and noodles are popular choices in various cuisines worldwide, offering endless possibilities for creative and wholesome cooking.

Cabbage

This Eastern Europe staple is a true wonder food. There are only 33 calories in a cup of cooked shredded cabbage, and it retains all its nutritional goodness no matter how long you cook it. Eating cabbage raw (18 calories per shredded cup), cooked, as sauerkraut (27 calories per drained cup), or coleslaw (calories depend on dressing) only once a week is enough to protect against colon cancer.

And it may be a longevity-enhancing food. Surveys in the United States, Greece, and Japan show that people who eat a lot of it have the least colon cancer and the lowest death rates overall.

Nutritional Profile:

Cabbage is celebrated for its exceptional nutritional density, offering an impressive array of vitamins, minerals, antioxidants, and dietary fiber. A single cup (about 89 grams) of chopped cabbage provides:

Vitamin C: Cabbage is a rich source of vitamin C, a potent antioxidant that supports immune function, collagen synthesis, and wound healing.

Vitamin K: Essential for blood clotting and bone health, vitamin K is abundant in cabbage, contributing to overall skeletal integrity.

Fiber: Cabbage is high in fiber, promoting digestive health, regulating blood sugar levels, and supporting weight management.

Potassium: Crucial for heart health and electrolyte balance, potassium is found in cabbage in significant amounts.

Folate: Important for DNA synthesis and cell division, folate is present in cabbage, contributing to overall cellular function.

Phytochemicals: Cabbage contains various phytochemicals, including sulforaphane, indole-3-carbinol, and glucosinolates, which have potent antioxidant and anti-inflammatory properties.

Cancer Prevention Properties:

One of the most extensively studied health benefits of cabbage is its potential to reduce the risk of certain types of cancer. Cruciferous vegetables like cabbage contain bioactive compounds, such as sulforaphane and indole-3-carbinol, which have been shown to:

Inhibit the growth and proliferation of cancer cells.

Induce apoptosis (programmed cell death) in malignant cells.

Detoxify carcinogens and enhance their excretion from the body.

Suppress the formation of tumors in animal models.

Modulate gene expression and signaling pathways involved in cancer development and progression.

Digestive Health Benefits:

Cabbage is rich in fiber, both soluble and insoluble, which supports digestive health and prevents constipation. The fiber in cabbage adds bulk to stool, promotes regular bowel movements, and nourishes beneficial gut bacteria, contributing to a healthy gut microbiome. Additionally, cabbage contains compounds like glucosinolates, which have been associated with a reduced risk of gastrointestinal cancers, including colorectal cancer.

Anti-inflammatory and Antioxidant Properties:

Chronic inflammation and oxidative stress are underlying factors in the development of numerous chronic diseases, including cardiovascular disorders, diabetes, and neurodegenerative conditions. Cabbage contains a diverse range of antioxidants and anti-inflammatory compounds, such as vitamin C, sulforaphane, and anthocyanins, which help:

Neutralize free radicals and prevent oxidative damage to cells and tissues.

Suppress pro-inflammatory cytokines and enzymes, reducing systemic inflammation.

Protect against age-related cognitive decline and neurodegenerative diseases, such as Alzheimer's disease and Parkinson's disease.

Heart Health Promotion:

Incorporating cabbage into your diet may have beneficial effects on cardiovascular health, thanks to its rich nutrient content and bioactive compounds. Cabbage consumption has been associated with:

Lowering LDL cholesterol levels and improving the ratio of HDL to LDL cholesterol, reducing the risk of atherosclerosis and heart disease.

Decreasing blood pressure levels and promoting vasodilation, helps maintain healthy blood pressure and vascular function.

Inhibiting platelet aggregation and thrombus formation, reducing the risk of blood clots and cardiovascular events like heart attacks and strokes.

Weight Management Support:

Cabbage is a low-calorie, nutrient-dense food that can be a valuable addition to weight management efforts. Its high fiber content promotes satiety and reduces hunger, helping to control calorie intake and prevent overeating. Additionally, cabbage is low in fat and carbohydrates, making it an excellent choice for individuals seeking to maintain a healthy weight and improve overall dietary quality.

Skin Health Enhancement:

The abundance of vitamin C and other antioxidants in cabbage makes it beneficial for skin health and appearance. Vitamin C is essential for collagen synthesis, the protein responsible for maintaining skin elasticity and firmness. Additionally, antioxidants help protect the skin from oxidative damage caused by UV radiation and environmental pollutants, reducing the risk of premature aging, wrinkles, and skin cancer.

Versatile Culinary Uses:

Cabbage is a highly versatile ingredient that can be enjoyed in various culinary preparations, from raw salads and coleslaws to soups, stews, stir-fries, and fermented dishes like sauerkraut and kimchi. Its mild flavor and crunchy texture make it a popular choice for adding bulk, nutrition, and flavor to meals, while its long shelf life and affordability make it accessible to a wide range of consumers.

Carrots

What list of health-promoting, fat-fighting foods would be complete without Bugs Bunny's favorite? A medium-sized carrot carries about 55 calories and is a nutritional powerhouse. The orange color comes from beta-carotene, a powerful cancer-preventing nutrient (provitamin A).

Chop and toss them with pasta, grate them into rice, or add them to a stir-fry. Combine them with parsnips, oranges, raisins, lemon juice, chicken, potatoes, broccoli, or lamb to create flavorful dishes. Spice them with tarragon, dill, cinnamon or nutmeg. Add finely chopped carrots to soups and spaghetti sauce – they impart a natural sweetness without adding sugar.

Nutritional Profile:

Carrots are celebrated for their exceptional nutritional density, offering a wide array of essential nutrients in a low-calorie package. A single medium-sized carrot (about 61 grams) provides:

Vitamin A: Carrots are rich in beta-carotene, a precursor to vitamin A, which is essential for vision, immune function, and skin health.

Vitamin K1: Crucial for blood clotting and bone metabolism, vitamin K1 is present in carrots, contributing to overall skeletal health.

Vitamin C: A potent antioxidant, vitamin C supports immune function, collagen synthesis, and wound healing, all of which are important for overall health and well-being.

Fiber: Carrots are a good source of dietary fiber, which promotes digestive health, regulates blood sugar levels, and supports weight management.

Potassium: Important for heart health and muscle function, potassium is found in carrots, contributing to overall cardiovascular and muscular health.

Eye Health Promotion:

One of the most well-known benefits of carrots is their role in promoting eye health and vision. Carrots are rich in beta-carotene, a type of carotenoid that is converted into vitamin A in the body. Vitamin A is essential for the synthesis of rhodopsin, a pigment in the retina that is crucial for low-light and color vision. Regular consumption of carrots may help:

Maintain healthy vision and prevent age-related macular degeneration (AMD), a leading cause of vision loss in older adults.

Protect the eyes from oxidative damage caused by exposure to UV radiation and harmful environmental pollutants.

Support overall eye health and function, reducing the risk of cataracts and other eye disorders associated with aging.

Antioxidant Properties:

Carrots are rich in antioxidants, including beta-carotene, lutein, zeaxanthin, and vitamin C, which help neutralize free radicals and prevent oxidative damage to cells and tissues. These antioxidants play a crucial role in:

Protecting against chronic diseases, including cardiovascular disorders, cancer, and neurodegenerative conditions.

Supporting immune function and reducing the risk of infections and inflammatory diseases.

Enhancing skin health and appearance by reducing oxidative stress and promoting collagen synthesis.

Heart Health Support:

Incorporating carrots into your diet may have beneficial effects on cardiovascular health, thanks to their nutrient content and antioxidant properties. Carrots have been associated with:

Lowering LDL cholesterol levels and improving the ratio of HDL to LDL cholesterol, reducing the risk of atherosclerosis and heart disease.

Decreasing blood pressure levels and promoting vasodilation, helps maintain healthy blood pressure and vascular function.

Inhibiting platelet aggregation and thrombus formation, reducing the risk of blood clots and cardiovascular events like heart attacks and strokes.

Digestive Health Benefits:

Carrots are a good source of dietary fiber, which supports digestive health and prevents constipation. The fiber in carrots adds bulk to stool, promotes regular bowel movements, and nourishes beneficial gut bacteria, contributing to a healthy gut microbiome. Additionally, carrots contain compounds like pectin, which may help regulate blood sugar levels and improve insulin sensitivity, reducing the risk of type 2 diabetes and metabolic syndrome.

Weight Management Support:

Due to their low calorie and high fiber content, carrots can be a valuable addition to weight management efforts. Incorporating carrots into meals and snacks can help promote satiety, reduce hunger, and prevent overeating. Additionally, carrots are naturally low in fat and carbohydrates, making them a nutritious and satisfying option for individuals seeking to maintain a healthy weight and improve overall dietary quality.

Skin Health Enhancement:

The abundance of beta-carotene and other antioxidants in carrots makes them beneficial for skin health and appearance. Beta-carotene is converted into vitamin A in the body, which is essential for maintaining healthy skin, reducing inflammation, and promoting collagen synthesis. Additionally, antioxidants help protect the skin from oxidative damage caused by UV radiation and environmental pollutants, reducing the risk of premature aging, wrinkles, and skin cancer.

Versatile Culinary Uses:

Carrots are a highly versatile vegetable that can be enjoyed in various culinary preparations, both raw and cooked. From salads and slaws to soups, stews, stir-fries, and juices, carrots add color, flavor, and nutritional value to a wide range of dishes. Their natural sweetness makes them a popular ingredient in both savory and sweet recipes, while their crunchy texture adds texture and substance to meals.

Chicken

White meat contains 245 calories per four-ounce serving and dark meat, 285. It's an excellent source of protein, iron, niacin and zinc. Skinned chicken is healthiest, but most experts recommend waiting until after cooking to remove it because the skin keeps the meat moist during cooking.

Nutritional Profile:

Chicken is renowned for its high protein content, making it a staple in many athletes and fitness enthusiasts' diets. A 100-gram serving of skinless, boneless chicken breast provides approximately 31 grams of protein, making it an excellent source of this vital macronutrient. Protein is crucial for muscle repair and growth, making chicken an ideal choice for individuals looking to build or maintain muscle mass.

In addition to protein, chicken is also rich in various vitamins and minerals essential for overall health. It contains significant amounts of vitamins B6 and B12, which play crucial roles in energy metabolism and red blood cell formation. Furthermore, chicken is a good source of niacin, a B vitamin important for DNA repair and cellular function.

Minerals such as phosphorus, selenium, and zinc are also abundant in chicken. Phosphorus is vital for bone health and energy production, while selenium acts as a powerful antioxidant, protecting cells from oxidative damage. Zinc is essential for immune function, wound healing, and protein synthesis, further enhancing the nutritional value of chicken.

Health Benefits:

Muscle Development and Repair:

Chicken's high protein content provides the necessary amino acids for muscle repair and growth.

Consuming chicken post-exercise helps replenish protein stores, aiding in muscle recovery.

Weight Management:

The lean protein in chicken helps increase satiety, reducing overall calorie intake.

Incorporating chicken into a balanced diet can support weight loss and weight management efforts.

Heart Health:

Chicken is low in saturated fat and cholesterol, making it a heart-healthy protein choice.

The niacin and B vitamins in chicken contribute to healthy cholesterol levels, reducing the risk of cardiovascular disease.

Immune Support:

Chicken contains selenium and zinc, which play key roles in immune function.

Regular consumption of chicken may help strengthen the immune system and enhance resistance to infections.

Bone Health:

The phosphorus content in chicken supports bone health and skeletal strength.

Including chicken in the diet can contribute to the prevention of osteoporosis and bone fractures.

Blood Sugar Regulation:

The protein in chicken helps stabilize blood sugar levels, reducing the risk of insulin spikes.

Incorporating chicken into meals can aid in blood sugar management, particularly for individuals with diabetes.

Cognitive Function:

The B vitamins in chicken, particularly B6 and B12, support neurological function and cognitive health.

Regular consumption of chicken may help maintain brain health and reduce the risk of cognitive decline with age.

Cooking Tips and Considerations:

While chicken offers numerous health benefits, it's essential to consider cooking methods and portion sizes to maximize its nutritional value. Here are some tips for preparing and enjoying chicken:

Choose lean cuts: Opt for skinless, boneless chicken breasts or thighs to minimize saturated fat intake.

Avoid frying: Instead of frying chicken, try healthier cooking methods such as baking, grilling, or sautéing.

Use herbs and spices: Enhance the flavor of chicken dishes with herbs, spices, and marinades instead of relying on excess salt or high-calorie sauces.

Practice portion control: Be mindful of portion sizes to avoid consuming excess calories and maintain a balanced diet.

Incorporate variety: Experiment with different chicken recipes and cooking techniques to keep meals exciting and nutritious.

Corn

It's a grain – not a vegetable – and is another food that's gotten a bum rap. People think it has little to offer nutritionally and that just isn't so. There are 178 calories in a cup of cooked kernels. It contains good amounts of iron, zinc, and potassium, and University of Nebraska researchers say it delivers a high-quality protein, too.

The Tarahumara Indians of Mexico eat corn, beans, and hardly anything else. Virgil Brown, M.D., of Mount Sinai School of Medicine in New York, points out that high blood cholesterol and cardiovascular heart disease are almost nonexistent among them.

Nutritional Composition:

Corn is a nutrient-rich grain that serves as a significant source of energy and essential nutrients. It contains carbohydrates, primarily in the form of starch, which provides a steady supply of energy to the body. Additionally, corn is rich in dietary fiber, with both soluble and insoluble fibers playing vital roles in digestive health and overall wellness.

One of the key nutritional components of corn is its vitamin content. It contains significant amounts of vitamins A, B vitamins (including thiamine, niacin, and folate), and vitamin C. These vitamins are essential for various bodily functions, including vision health, energy metabolism, and immune function.

Furthermore, corn is a good source of minerals such as magnesium, phosphorus, and potassium. These minerals play critical roles in bone health, muscle function, and electrolyte balance within the body. Additionally, corn contains antioxidants such as lutein and zeaxanthin, which contribute to eye health and may help protect against age-related macular degeneration.

Health Benefits:

Digestive Health:

The fiber content in corn promotes regular bowel movements and prevents constipation.

Soluble fiber in corn helps regulate blood sugar levels and may reduce the risk of developing type 2 diabetes.

Heart Health:

The soluble fiber and antioxidants in corn can help lower cholesterol levels and reduce the risk of heart disease.

Potassium in corn helps regulate blood pressure, promoting cardiovascular health.

Weight Management:

The fiber and complex carbohydrates in corn help increase satiety and prevent overeating.

Incorporating corn into a balanced diet may aid in weight loss and weight management efforts.

Eye Health:

Corn is rich in lutein and zeaxanthin, antioxidants that protect against age-related macular degeneration and cataracts.

Regular consumption of corn may help maintain vision health and prevent eye disorders.

Energy Boost:

The carbohydrates in corn provide a readily available source of energy for physical activity and cognitive function.

Corn-based snacks can serve as convenient energy-boosting options for individuals on the go.

Skin Health:

The vitamin A content in corn supports healthy skin by promoting cell turnover and repair.

Including corn in the diet may contribute to a radiant complexion and overall skin health.

Cancer Prevention:

The antioxidants in corn, including lutein, zeaxanthin, and ferulic acid, possess anticancer properties.

Regular consumption of corn may help reduce the risk of certain types of cancer, including colon cancer.

Cooking Tips and Considerations:

While corn offers numerous health benefits, it's essential to consider cooking methods and preparation techniques to maximize its nutritional value. Here are some tips for incorporating corn into a healthy diet:

Choose whole corn: Opt for fresh, whole corn kernels or frozen corn over canned varieties, which may contain added sodium and preservatives.

Steam or boil: Cooking corn using methods such as steaming or boiling helps preserve its nutritional content while minimizing added fats and calories.

Add variety: Experiment with different corn-based dishes, including salads, soups, stir-fries, and casseroles, to enjoy its versatility and flavor.

Avoid excessive processing: Limit consumption of highly processed corn products, such as corn chips and corn syrup, which may contain added sugars, unhealthy fats, and artificial ingredients.

Balance with other foods: Incorporate corn into balanced meals that include a variety of nutrient-rich foods, such as lean protein, whole grains, vegetables, and healthy fats.

Cottage Cheese

As long as we're talking about losing weight and fat-fighting foods, we had to mention cottage cheese.

Low-fat (2%) cottage cheese has 205 calories per cup and is admirably low in fat while providing respectable amounts of calcium and the B vitamin riboflavin. Season with spices such as dill, or garden fresh vegetables such as scallions and chives for extra zip.

To make it sweeter, add raisins or one of the fruit spreads with no sugar added. You can also use cottage cheese in cooking, baking, fillings, and dips where you would otherwise use sour cream or cream cheese.

Nutritional Composition:

Cottage cheese is a nutrient-rich dairy product made from curdled milk, offering a wealth of essential nutrients in each serving. Its nutritional profile includes:

Protein: Cottage cheese is renowned for its high protein content, making it a favorite among fitness enthusiasts and individuals seeking to increase their protein intake. A typical serving of cottage cheese provides approximately 25 grams of protein, making it an excellent source of this vital macronutrient. Protein is essential for muscle repair, growth, and overall tissue maintenance.

Calcium: Cottage cheese is rich in calcium, a mineral crucial for bone health, muscle function, and nerve transmission. A single serving of cottage cheese can supply up to 20% of the recommended daily intake of calcium, making it an excellent choice for maintaining strong and healthy bones.

Phosphorus: Alongside calcium, cottage cheese contains phosphorus, another essential mineral vital for bone formation and maintenance. Phosphorus works synergistically with calcium to support skeletal health and ensure proper mineralization of bones and teeth.

Vitamin B12: Cottage cheese is a good source of vitamin B12, a water-soluble vitamin essential for nerve function, red blood cell production, and DNA synthesis. Adequate intake of vitamin B12 is crucial for maintaining overall health and preventing deficiencies associated with fatigue, weakness, and neurological disorders.

Riboflavin (Vitamin B2): Cottage cheese contains riboflavin, a B vitamin involved in energy metabolism, cellular growth, and antioxidant defense. Riboflavin plays a vital role in converting food into energy and supporting various physiological processes within the body.

Other Nutrients: Cottage cheese also provides significant amounts of other essential nutrients, including phosphorus, selenium, potassium, and zinc, contributing to overall health and well-being.

Health Benefits:

Muscle Development and Recovery:

The high-quality protein in cottage cheese provides essential amino acids necessary for muscle repair, growth, and recovery.

Consuming cottage cheese post-exercise can help replenish protein stores and support muscle recovery.

Bone Health:

The calcium and phosphorus in cottage cheese play crucial roles in maintaining strong and healthy bones.

Regular consumption of cottage cheese may help reduce the risk of osteoporosis and bone fractures, particularly in older adults.

Weight Management:

Cottage cheese is low in calories and rich in protein, making it a satisfying and nutritious option for individuals seeking to manage their weight.

The protein and calcium in cottage cheese help promote feelings of fullness and satiety, reducing overall calorie intake.

Digestive Health:

Cottage cheese contains probiotics, beneficial bacteria that promote gut health and digestion.

The probiotics in cottage cheese may help improve digestion, alleviate symptoms of irritable bowel syndrome (IBS), and support a healthy gut microbiome.

Cardiovascular Health:

The calcium and potassium in cottage cheese support cardiovascular health by regulating blood pressure and promoting heart function.

Consuming cottage cheese as part of a balanced diet may help lower the risk of hypertension and cardiovascular disease.

Immune Support:

Cottage cheese contains vitamins and minerals, including vitamin B12, zinc, and selenium, which support immune function and enhance the body's defense against infections.

Including cottage cheese in the diet may help strengthen the immune system and reduce the risk of illness.

Skin and Hair Health:

The protein, vitamin B12, and zinc in cottage cheese contribute to healthy skin and hair growth.

Regular consumption of cottage cheese may help maintain radiant skin, strong nails, and lustrous hair.

Cooking Tips and Considerations:

Incorporating cottage cheese into your diet is simple and versatile, allowing for a wide range of culinary possibilities. Here are some tips for enjoying cottage cheese:

Enjoy it plain: Enjoy cottage cheese on its own as a quick and nutritious snack, or pair it with fresh fruits, vegetables, or whole grain crackers for added flavor and texture.

Use it in recipes: Incorporate cottage cheese into various recipes, including smoothies, salads, dips, sauces, and baked goods, to enhance their nutritional value and creaminess.

Mix with herbs and spices: Add flavor to cottage cheese by mixing in herbs, spices, or condiments such as black pepper, chives, garlic powder, or hot sauce.

Include it in savory dishes: Use cottage cheese as a substitute for ricotta or cream cheese in savory dishes such as lasagna, stuffed pasta, or savory pancakes.

Blend into smoothies: Blend cottage cheese into smoothies or shakes to add creaminess, protein, and nutrients without altering the flavor significantly.

Figs

Fiber-rich figs are low in calories at 37 per medium (2.25" diameter) raw fig and 48 per dried fig. A recent study by the USDA demonstrated that they contribute to a feeling of fullness and prevent overeating. Subjects complained of being asked to eat too much food when fed a diet containing more figs than a similar diet with an identical number of calories.

Serve them with other fruits and cheeses. Or poach them in fruit juice and serve them warm or cold. You can stuff them with mild white cheese or puree them to use as a filling for cookies and low-calorie pastries.

Nutritional Composition:

Figs are nutrient-dense fruits that provide a concentrated source of essential vitamins, minerals, and dietary fiber. A single serving of figs (about 3-4 medium-sized fruits) typically contains the following nutrients:

Fiber: Figs are particularly rich in dietary fiber, with both soluble and insoluble fibers present in abundance. Fiber promotes digestive health by supporting regular bowel movements, preventing constipation, and aiding in the removal of waste and toxins from the body.

Vitamins: Figs are a good source of various vitamins, including vitamin A, vitamin B6, vitamin K, and vitamin C. These vitamins play critical roles in immune function, vision health, blood clotting, and collagen production, among other essential bodily processes.

Minerals: Figs contain essential minerals such as potassium, calcium, magnesium, and iron. Potassium helps regulate blood pressure and maintain proper fluid balance in the body, while calcium and magnesium support bone health and muscle function. Iron is necessary for red blood cell formation and oxygen transport.

Antioxidants: Figs are rich in polyphenols, flavonoids, and other antioxidants that help protect cells from oxidative damage caused by free radicals. These antioxidants have anti-inflammatory properties and may help reduce the risk of chronic diseases such as heart disease, cancer, and neurodegenerative disorders.

Health Benefits:

Digestive Health:

The high fiber content in figs promotes regular bowel movements and relieves constipation.

Figs contain prebiotics, which nourish beneficial gut bacteria and support a healthy gut microbiome.

Heart Health:

The potassium and fiber in figs help regulate blood pressure and cholesterol levels, reducing the risk of heart disease.

Figs contain antioxidants that protect against oxidative stress and inflammation, which are implicated in cardiovascular diseases.

Bone Health:

Figs are rich in calcium, magnesium, and vitamin K, essential nutrients for maintaining strong and healthy bones.

Regular consumption of figs may help prevent osteoporosis and reduce the risk of fractures and bone-related disorders.

Blood Sugar Control:

The soluble fiber in figs slows down the absorption of glucose in the bloodstream, helping to stabilize blood sugar levels.

Figs have a low glycemic index, making them a suitable option for individuals with diabetes or those seeking to manage blood sugar levels.

Weight Management:

The fiber and low-calorie content of figs promote feelings of fullness and satiety, reducing overall calorie intake.

Including figs in a balanced diet may help support weight loss and weight management efforts.

Skin Health:

The vitamin A and antioxidants in figs help protect the skin from oxidative damage and promote a healthy complexion.

Figs contain compounds that may have anti-aging effects and help reduce the appearance of wrinkles and fine lines.

Cancer Prevention:

The antioxidants and phytochemicals in figs have been associated with a reduced risk of certain types of cancer, including breast, colon, and prostate cancer.

Figs contain compounds that inhibit the growth and proliferation of cancer cells and promote apoptosis (programmed cell death).

Cooking Tips and Considerations:

Figs can be enjoyed fresh, dried, or in various culinary preparations, making them a versatile and delicious addition to meals and snacks. Here are some tips for incorporating figs into your diet:

Fresh Figs: Enjoy ripe figs on their own as a nutritious snack, or add them to salads, yogurt parfaits, or cheese platters for a touch of natural sweetness and flavor.

Dried Figs: Use dried figs in baking recipes such as muffins, cakes, and bread, or incorporate them into granola bars, trail mixes, and oatmeal for added texture and sweetness.

Fig Jam: Make homemade fig jam or preserves to spread on toast, crackers, or sandwiches, or use it as a topping for pancakes, waffles, or yogurt.

Stuffed Figs: Stuff fresh figs with cheese, nuts, or honey for a simple yet elegant appetizer or dessert option.

Fig Sauce: Blend fresh or dried figs with water or citrus juice to make a flavorful sauce or dressing for salads, meats, or roasted vegetables.

Fish

The health benefits of fish are greater than experts imagined – and they've always considered it a healthy food.

The calorie count in the average four-ounce serving of a deep-sea fish runs from a low of 90 calories in abalone to a high of 236 in herring. Water-packed tuna, for example, has 154 calories. It's hard to gain weight eating seafood.

As far back as 1985, articles in the New England Journal of Medicine showed a clear link between eating fish regularly and lower rates of heart disease. The reason is that oils in fish thin the blood, reduce blood pressure, and lower cholesterol.

Nutritional Composition:

Fish is a nutrient-rich food that offers a plethora of essential nutrients crucial for optimal health and well-being. Its nutritional profile varies depending on the species, but in general, fish is an excellent source of:

Protein: Fish is rich in high-quality protein, containing all the essential amino acids necessary for muscle repair, growth, and maintenance. Protein is also vital for supporting various physiological functions, including enzyme production, hormone regulation, and immune function.

Omega-3 Fatty Acids: Fatty fish such as salmon, mackerel, trout, and sardines are particularly rich in omega-3 fatty acids, including eicosapentaenoic acid (EPA) and docosahexaenoic acid (DHA). These essential fatty acids play critical roles in brain health, cardiovascular function, inflammation regulation, and cognitive function.

Vitamins: Fish is a significant source of various vitamins, including vitamin D, vitamin B12, and vitamin A. Vitamin D is essential for bone health, immune function, and calcium absorption, while vitamin B12 is necessary for red blood cell formation, nerve function, and DNA synthesis. Vitamin A supports vision health, immune function, and skin integrity.

Minerals: Fish provides essential minerals such as iodine, selenium, zinc, and iron. Iodine is crucial for thyroid function and hormone regulation, while selenium acts as a powerful antioxidant, protecting cells from oxidative damage. Zinc is necessary for immune function, wound healing, and protein synthesis, while iron is vital for oxygen transport and energy production.

Health Benefits:

Cardiovascular Health:

Omega-3 fatty acids in fish help reduce triglyceride levels, lower blood pressure, and prevent the formation of blood clots, reducing the risk of heart disease and stroke.

Consuming fish regularly is associated with a lower incidence of cardiovascular events and improved heart health outcomes.

Brain Function and Cognitive Health:

Omega-3 fatty acids, particularly DHA, are essential for brain development, cognitive function, and memory retention.

Regular fish consumption has been linked to a reduced risk of age-related cognitive decline, Alzheimer's disease, and other neurodegenerative disorders.

Eye Health:

The omega-3 fatty acids EPA and DHA are critical for maintaining vision health and reducing the risk of age-related macular degeneration and cataracts.

Including fish in the diet may help protect against eye disorders and preserve visual acuity as we age.

Inflammation Reduction:

Omega-3 fatty acids possess anti-inflammatory properties that help alleviate inflammation and reduce the risk of chronic inflammatory conditions such as arthritis, asthma, and inflammatory bowel disease.

Consuming fish regularly may help modulate the body's inflammatory response and promote overall health and well-being.

Immune Support:

The protein, vitamins, and minerals in fish support immune function and enhance the body's ability to fight off infections and illnesses.

Including fish in the diet can help strengthen the immune system and improve resilience to common pathogens.

Bone Health:

Vitamin D and calcium in fish contribute to bone health and density, reducing the risk of osteoporosis and fractures.

Consuming fish regularly, especially fatty fish, can help maintain strong and healthy bones throughout life.

Weight Management:

The high protein content and low-calorie nature of fish make it a satiating and nutrient-dense food choice for individuals seeking to manage their weight.

Incorporating fish into a balanced diet can help promote feelings of fullness, reduce calorie intake, and support weight loss and weight maintenance efforts.

Cooking Tips and Considerations:

Enjoying fish as part of a healthy diet is simple and versatile, offering endless culinary possibilities. Here are some tips for incorporating fish into your meals:

Choose a Variety of Species: Experiment with different types of fish, including salmon, tuna, mackerel, trout, sardines, and haddock, to enjoy a diverse range of flavors and nutritional benefits.

Opt for Healthy Cooking Methods: Grill, bake, broil, or steam fish instead of frying to minimize added fats and calories while preserving its natural flavor and nutrients.

Enhance with Herbs and Spices: Season fish with herbs, spices, citrus zest, or marinades to add depth of flavor without excessive salt or added calories.

Include Fish in Balanced Meals: Serve fish alongside a variety of vegetables, whole grains, and legumes to create well-rounded and nutritious meals that support overall health and wellness.

Be Mindful of Sustainability: Choose fish that are sustainably sourced and harvested to minimize environmental impact and support responsible fishing practices.

Dr. Joel Kremer, at Albany Medical College in New York, discovered that daily supplements of fish oil brought dramatic relief to the inflammation and stiff joints of rheumatoid arthritis.

Greens

We're talking collard, chicory, beet, kale, mustard, Swiss chard and turnip greens. They all belong to the same family as spinach, and that's one of the super-stars. No matter how hard you try, you can't load a cup of plain cooked greens with any more than 50 calories.

They're full of fiber, loaded with vitamins A and C, and free of fat. You can use them in salads, soups, casseroles, or any dish where you would normally use spinach.

Nutritional Composition:

Greens are nutrient-dense powerhouses packed with an impressive array of vitamins, minerals, antioxidants, and phytonutrients. While the exact nutritional profile varies among different types of greens, they typically contain the following key nutrients:

Vitamins: Greens are rich in various vitamins, including vitamin A, vitamin C, vitamin K, and several B vitamins such as folate (vitamin B9). Vitamin A supports vision health, immune function, and skin integrity, while vitamin C acts as an antioxidant, boosting immunity and collagen production. Vitamin K plays a crucial role in blood clotting and bone health, while folate is essential for DNA synthesis and cell division.

Minerals: Greens provide an abundance of minerals, including calcium, magnesium, potassium, iron, and manganese. Calcium is vital for bone health and muscle function, while magnesium supports nerve transmission and muscle relaxation. Potassium helps regulate blood pressure and fluid balance, while iron is necessary for oxygen transport and energy production. Manganese acts as a cofactor for various enzymes involved in metabolism and antioxidant defense.

Dietary Fiber: Greens are an excellent source of dietary fiber, including both soluble and insoluble fibers. Fiber promotes digestive health by supporting regular bowel movements, preventing constipation, and nourishing beneficial gut bacteria. It also helps regulate blood sugar levels, reduce cholesterol levels, and promote feelings of fullness and satiety.

Antioxidants: Greens are rich in antioxidants such as beta-carotene, lutein, zeaxanthin, and flavonoids, which help neutralize harmful free radicals and reduce oxidative stress in the body. These antioxidants have anti-inflammatory properties and may help protect against chronic diseases such as heart disease, cancer, and neurodegenerative disorders.

Health Benefits:

Heart Health:

The potassium, magnesium, and fiber in greens help regulate blood pressure, reduce cholesterol levels, and support cardiovascular function.

Regular consumption of greens is associated with a lower risk of heart disease, stroke, and other cardiovascular events.

Bone Health:

The calcium, vitamin K, and magnesium in greens support bone health and density, reducing the risk of osteoporosis and fractures.

Including greens in the diet may help maintain strong and healthy bones throughout life, particularly in older adults.

Digestive Health:

The dietary fiber in greens promotes regular bowel movements, relieves constipation, and supports a healthy gut microbiome.

Greens contain prebiotics, which nourish beneficial gut bacteria and improve digestive function.

Immune Support:

The vitamins, minerals, and antioxidants in greens support immune function and enhance the body's defense against infections and illnesses.

Including greens in the diet may help strengthen the immune system and reduce the risk of common colds, flu, and other respiratory infections.

Weight Management:

The low-calorie and high-fiber content of greens makes them a nutrient-dense and satiating food choice for individuals seeking to manage their weight.

Incorporating greens into meals and snacks can help promote feelings of fullness, reduce calorie intake, and support weight loss and weight maintenance efforts.

Eye Health:

The antioxidants lutein and zeaxanthin, found in greens such as spinach and kale, promote vision health and reduce the risk of age-related macular degeneration and cataracts.

Regular consumption of greens may help protect against eye disorders and preserve visual acuity.

Skin Health:

The vitamins A and C, as well as antioxidants such as beta-carotene, in greens, support skin health by promoting collagen production, reducing oxidative stress, and preventing premature aging.

Including greens in the diet may help maintain a radiant complexion and healthy skin.

Cooking Tips and Considerations:

Incorporating greens into meals and snacks is simple and versatile, offering endless culinary possibilities. Here are some tips for enjoying greens:

Enjoy Raw or Cooked: Greens can be enjoyed raw in salads, wraps, and smoothies, or cooked in stir-fries, soups, stews, and sautés.

Mix and Match: Combine different types of greens to create flavorful and nutritious salads, side dishes, and main courses.

Add to Smoothies: Blend greens such as spinach, kale, or Swiss chard into smoothies or juices for an added nutrient boost.

Use as Wraps: Use large leaves of greens such as collard greens or Swiss chard as wraps or taco shells filled with vegetables, proteins, and healthy spreads.

Enhance with Herbs and Spices: Season cooked greens with herbs, spices, garlic, onions, citrus juice, or vinegar to add flavor and depth to dishes.

Experiment with Recipes: Explore new recipes and cooking techniques to discover creative ways to incorporate greens into your meals and snacks.

Kiwi

This New Zealand native is a sweet treat at only 46 calories per fruit. Chinese public health officials praise the tasty fruit for its high vitamin C content and potassium. It is stored easily in the refrigerator for up to a month. Most people like it peeled, but the fuzzy skin is also edible.

Nutritional Composition:

Kiwi is a nutritional powerhouse, packed with essential nutrients that contribute to overall health and well-being. A single serving of kiwi (approximately one medium fruit) typically contains the following nutrients:

Vitamin C: Kiwi is one of the richest sources of vitamin C, containing more than twice the amount found in oranges. Vitamin C is a powerful antioxidant that supports immune function, collagen synthesis, and wound healing. It also helps protect cells from oxidative damage and promotes healthy skin, gums, and teeth.

Fiber: Kiwi is high in dietary fiber, including both soluble and insoluble fibers. Fiber promotes digestive health by regulating bowel movements, preventing constipation, and supporting the growth of beneficial gut bacteria. It also helps regulate blood sugar levels, lower cholesterol, and promote satiety.

Vitamin K: Kiwi contains vitamin K, a fat-soluble vitamin essential for blood clotting, bone metabolism, and cardiovascular health. Vitamin K also plays a role in maintaining strong and healthy bones, preventing osteoporosis, and reducing the risk of fractures.

Potassium: Kiwi is a good source of potassium, an essential mineral that helps regulate blood pressure, fluid balance, and muscle function. Potassium also supports cardiovascular health by counteracting the effects of sodium and reducing the risk of hypertension and stroke.

Antioxidants: Kiwi is rich in antioxidants such as flavonoids, polyphenols, and carotenoids, which help neutralize free radicals and protect cells from oxidative damage. These antioxidants have anti-inflammatory properties and may help reduce the risk of chronic diseases such as heart disease, cancer, and neurodegenerative disorders.

Health Benefits:

Immune Support:

The high vitamin C content in kiwi strengthens the immune system and enhances the body's defense against infections and illnesses.

Regular consumption of kiwi may help reduce the severity and duration of colds, flu, and other respiratory infections.

Digestive Health:

The fiber in kiwi promotes regular bowel movements, prevents constipation, and supports a healthy gut microbiome.

Kiwi contains enzymes such as actinidin, which aid in the digestion of proteins and may help alleviate symptoms of indigestion and bloating.

Heart Health:

The potassium and fiber in kiwi help regulate blood pressure, reduce cholesterol levels, and support cardiovascular function.

Consuming kiwi as part of a heart-healthy diet may help lower the risk of heart disease, stroke, and other cardiovascular conditions.

Skin Health:

The vitamin C and antioxidants in kiwi promote collagen synthesis, skin regeneration, and protection against UV-induced damage.

Including kiwi in the diet may help maintain youthful skin, reduce the appearance of wrinkles and age spots, and protect against sunburn and skin cancer.

Eye Health:

Kiwi contains lutein and zeaxanthin, carotenoid antioxidants that support vision health and protect against age-related macular degeneration and cataracts.

Regular consumption of kiwi may help maintain visual acuity and reduce the risk of eye disorders associated with aging.

Weight Management:

The fiber and low-calorie content of kiwi make it a satisfying and nutrient-dense food choice for individuals seeking to manage their weight.

Incorporating kiwi into a balanced diet may help promote feelings of fullness, reduce calorie intake, and support weight loss and weight maintenance efforts.

Anti-Inflammatory Effects:

The antioxidants and phytochemicals in kiwi possess anti-inflammatory properties that help reduce inflammation and alleviate symptoms of inflammatory conditions such as arthritis and asthma.

Consuming kiwi regularly may help modulate the body's inflammatory response and promote overall health and well-being.

Cooking Tips and Considerations:

Kiwi is a versatile fruit that can be enjoyed in various ways, both fresh and cooked. Here are some tips for incorporating kiwi into your diet:

Fresh Consumption: Enjoy ripe kiwi on its own as a refreshing snack, or slice it and add it to fruit salads, yogurt parfaits, or smoothie bowls for added flavor and nutrition.

Desserts and Sweets: Use kiwi as a topping for desserts such as cakes, tarts, and pavlovas, or incorporate it into fruit salads, sorbets, and gelato for a burst of tropical flavor.

Savory Dishes: Add diced kiwi to savory dishes such as salsa, salads, ceviche, or grilled fish or chicken for a tangy and refreshing twist.

Beverages: Blend kiwi into smoothies, juices, or cocktails for a refreshing and nutritious beverage option, or infuse water with kiwi slices for a hint of flavor.

Preserve and Freeze: Make kiwi jam, chutney, or compote to enjoy year-round, or freeze-peeled kiwi slices for a refreshing frozen treat.

Leeks

These members of the onion family look like giant scallions and are every bit as healthful and flavorful as their better-known cousins. They come as close to calorie-free as they get at a mere 32 calories per cooked cup.

You can poach or broil halved leeks and then marinate them in vinaigrette or season with Romano cheese, fine mustard, or herbs. They also make a good soup.

Nutritional Composition:

Leeks are a nutrient-dense vegetable packed with vitamins, minerals, dietary fiber, and phytochemicals. A single serving of leeks (approximately 1 cup chopped) typically contains the following nutrients:

Vitamins: Leeks are an excellent source of vitamins, particularly vitamin K, vitamin A, and vitamin C. Vitamin K plays a crucial role in blood clotting and bone health, while vitamin A supports vision health, immune function, and skin integrity. Vitamin C is a potent antioxidant that boosts immune function, promotes collagen synthesis, and protects against oxidative damage.

Minerals: Leeks provide essential minerals such as manganese, folate, iron, and potassium. Manganese is necessary for enzyme activation and bone formation, while folate is crucial for DNA synthesis and cell division. Iron is vital for oxygen transport and energy production, while potassium helps regulate blood pressure and fluid balance.

Dietary Fiber: Leeks are rich in dietary fiber, including both soluble and insoluble fibers. Fiber promotes digestive health by preventing constipation, regulating bowel movements, and supporting the growth of beneficial gut bacteria. It also helps control blood sugar levels, lower cholesterol, and promote feelings of fullness.

Antioxidants: Leeks contain various antioxidants, including polyphenols, flavonoids, and sulfur compounds. These antioxidants help neutralize free radicals, reduce inflammation, and protect cells from oxidative damage. They also have anti-cancer properties and may help reduce the risk of chronic diseases such as heart disease, cancer, and neurodegenerative disorders.

Health Benefits:

Digestive Health:

The fiber in leeks promotes regular bowel movements, prevents constipation, and supports a healthy gut microbiome.

Leeks contain prebiotics, which nourish beneficial gut bacteria and improve digestive function.

Heart Health:

The antioxidants and sulfur compounds in leeks help lower cholesterol levels, reduce inflammation, and improve blood vessel function.

Consuming leeks as part of a heart-healthy diet may help reduce the risk of cardiovascular disease and stroke.

Bone Health:

The vitamin K and manganese in leeks support bone health and density, reducing the risk of osteoporosis and fractures.

Including leeks in the diet may help improve bone mineralization and prevent bone-related disorders.

Immune Support:

The vitamin C and antioxidants in leeks strengthen the immune system and enhance the body's defense against infections and illnesses.

Regular consumption of leeks may help reduce the severity and duration of colds, flu, and other respiratory infections.

Anti-Inflammatory Effects:

The antioxidants and sulfur compounds in leeks possess anti-inflammatory properties that help reduce inflammation and alleviate symptoms of inflammatory conditions such as arthritis and asthma.

Consuming leeks regularly may help modulate the body's inflammatory response and promote overall health and well-being.

Weight Management:

The fiber and low-calorie content of leeks makes them a satisfying and nutrient-dense food choice for individuals seeking to manage their weight.

Incorporating leeks into a balanced diet may help promote feelings of fullness, reduce calorie intake, and support weight loss and weight maintenance efforts.

Cancer Prevention:

The antioxidants and sulfur compounds in leeks have been associated with a reduced risk of certain types of cancer, including colon, prostate, and stomach cancer.

Consuming leeks as part of a plant-rich diet may help protect against cancer by reducing oxidative stress and inflammation.

Cooking Tips and Considerations:

Incorporating leeks into your diet is simple and versatile, offering endless culinary possibilities. Here are some tips for enjoying leeks:

Wash and Trim: Rinse leeks thoroughly under cold water to remove any dirt or debris trapped between the layers. Trim off the root end and dark green tops, leaving the white and light green portions for cooking.

Sauté or Roast: Sauté sliced leeks in olive oil or butter until tender and caramelized, or roast them alongside other vegetables for added flavor and texture.

Add to Soups and Stews: Chop leeks and add them to soups, stews, and broths for a mild onion flavor and nutrient boost. Leeks pair well with potatoes, carrots, celery, and herbs such as thyme and parsley.

Use as a Flavor Base: Use leeks as a flavor base for sauces, gravies, and stir-fries, similar to onions and garlic. Their subtle sweetness and aromatic flavor enhance the taste of savory dishes.

Grill or Broil: Cut leeks into large pieces, brush them with olive oil, and grill or broil until tender and charred for a smoky flavor and caramelized finish.

Lettuce

People think lettuce is nutritionally worthless, but nothing could be farther from the truth. You can't leave it out of your weight-loss plans, not at 10 calories per cup of raw romaine. It provides a lot of filling bulk for so few calories. And it's full of vitamin C, too. Go beyond iceberg lettuce with Boston, bibb, and cos varieties, or try watercress, arugula, radicchio, dandelion greens, purslane, and even parsley to liven up your salads.

Nutritional Composition:

Lettuce is a low-calorie vegetable that is packed with essential nutrients, including vitamins, minerals, and dietary fiber. A single serving of lettuce (approximately one cup shredded) typically contains the following nutrients:

Vitamins: Lettuce is rich in vitamins, particularly vitamin A, vitamin K, and vitamin C. Vitamin A is essential for vision health, immune function, and skin integrity. Vitamin K plays a crucial role in blood clotting and bone metabolism, while vitamin C is a potent antioxidant that supports immune function and collagen synthesis.

Minerals: Lettuce provides essential minerals such as potassium, manganese, and folate. Potassium helps regulate blood pressure and fluid balance, while manganese is necessary for enzyme activation and antioxidant defense. Folate is crucial for DNA synthesis and cell division, particularly during pregnancy.

Dietary Fiber: Lettuce is a good source of dietary fiber, including both soluble and insoluble fibers. Fiber promotes digestive health by regulating bowel movements, preventing constipation, and supporting a healthy gut microbiome. It also helps control blood sugar levels, lower cholesterol, and promote satiety.

Water: Lettuce has a high water content, which helps keep the body hydrated and supports overall hydration status. Adequate hydration is essential for various bodily functions, including temperature regulation, nutrient transport, and waste removal.

Health Benefits:

Weight Management:

Lettuce is low in calories and high in dietary fiber, making it a filling and nutritious food choice for individuals seeking to manage their weight.

Incorporating lettuce into meals and snacks can help increase satiety, reduce calorie intake, and support weight loss and weight maintenance efforts.

Digestive Health:

The fiber in lettuce promotes regular bowel movements, prevents constipation, and supports digestive health.

Lettuce contains water, which helps soften stool and alleviate symptoms of constipation.

Heart Health:

The potassium in lettuce helps regulate blood pressure and reduce the risk of hypertension and cardiovascular disease.

Consuming lettuce as part of a heart-healthy diet may help lower cholesterol levels and improve overall cardiovascular health.

Bone Health:

The vitamin K in lettuce plays a crucial role in bone metabolism and calcium absorption, supporting bone health and density.

Including lettuce in the diet may help reduce the risk of osteoporosis and fractures, particularly in older adults.

Immune Support:

The vitamin C and antioxidants in lettuce strengthen the immune system and enhance the body's defense against infections and illnesses.

Regular consumption of lettuce may help reduce the severity and duration of colds, flu, and other respiratory infections.

Skin Health:

The vitamin A and antioxidants in lettuce promote skin health by supporting collagen synthesis, reducing oxidative damage, and maintaining skin integrity.

Including lettuce in the diet may help prevent skin disorders and maintain a healthy complexion.

Hydration:

Lettuce has a high water content, which helps keep the body hydrated and supports overall hydration status.

Consuming lettuce, particularly in its raw form, can contribute to daily fluid intake and prevent dehydration.

Cooking Tips and Considerations:

Incorporating lettuce into your diet is simple and versatile, offering endless culinary possibilities. Here are some tips for enjoying lettuce:

Salad Base: Use lettuce as a base for salads, either on its own or mixed with other leafy greens and vegetables. Choose a variety of lettuce types, such as romaine, iceberg, leaf, or butterhead, for different flavors and textures.

Sandwich and Wrap Filling: Add lettuce leaves to sandwiches, wraps, burgers, and tacos for added crunch, moisture, and nutrition. Lettuce can also serve as a low-carb alternative to bread or tortillas in certain recipes.

Smoothie Ingredient: Blend lettuce leaves into smoothies or green juices for a nutritious boost without altering the flavor significantly. Lettuce pairs well with fruits, vegetables, herbs, and protein powders in smoothie recipes.

Stir-Fry Addition: Toss shredded lettuce into stir-fries or Asian-inspired dishes during the final minutes of cooking for a refreshing and crunchy texture. Lettuce can add volume and freshness to cooked dishes without adding excess calories or sodium.

Soup Garnish: Use lettuce leaves as a garnish for soups, stews, and curries to add color, texture, and a hint of freshness. Lettuce can be torn or shredded and added to hot dishes just before serving for a vibrant finishing touch.

Melons

Now, there's great taste and great nutrition in a low-calorie package! One cup of cantaloupe balls has 62 calories, one cup of casaba balls has 44 calories, one cup of honeydew balls has 62 calories and one cup of watermelon balls has 49 calories. They have some of the highest fiber content of any food and are delicious. Throw in handsome quantities of vitamins A and C plus a whopping 547 mg of potassium in that cup of cantaloupe, and you have a fat-burning health food beyond compare.

Nutritional Composition:

Melons are low-calorie fruits that are rich in essential nutrients, including vitamins, minerals, dietary fiber, and antioxidants. While the exact nutritional composition may vary depending on the specific variety of melon, a typical serving of melon (about one cup diced) contains the following nutrients:

Vitamins: Melons are an excellent source of various vitamins, particularly vitamin C, vitamin A, and vitamin K. Vitamin C is a potent antioxidant that supports immune function, collagen synthesis, and wound healing. Vitamin A is essential for vision health, immune function, and skin integrity, while vitamin K plays a crucial role in blood clotting and bone metabolism.

Minerals: Melons provide essential minerals such as potassium, magnesium, and folate. Potassium helps regulate blood pressure, fluid balance, and muscle function, while magnesium supports nerve function, muscle contraction, and bone health. Folate is necessary for DNA synthesis and cell division, particularly during pregnancy.

Dietary Fiber: Melons are a good source of dietary fiber, including both soluble and insoluble fibers. Fiber promotes digestive health by regulating bowel movements, preventing constipation, and supporting a healthy gut microbiome. It also helps control blood sugar levels, lower cholesterol, and promote feelings of fullness.

Water: Melons have a high water content, ranging from 85% to 95% depending on the variety. Adequate hydration is essential for various bodily functions, including temperature regulation, nutrient transport, and waste removal. Consuming melons can contribute to overall hydration status and help prevent dehydration.

Health Benefits:

Hydration:

Due to their high water content, melons are incredibly hydrating and can help maintain fluid balance within the body.

Consuming melons, particularly during hot weather or after physical activity, can help prevent dehydration and promote overall hydration status.

Immune Support:

The vitamin C and antioxidants in melons strengthen the immune system and enhance the body's defense against infections and illnesses.

Regular consumption of melons may help reduce the severity and duration of colds, flu, and other respiratory infections.

Heart Health:

The potassium and magnesium in melons help regulate blood pressure, reduce the risk of hypertension, and support cardiovascular health.

Consuming melons as part of a heart-healthy diet may help lower cholesterol levels, improve blood vessel function, and reduce the risk of heart disease and stroke.

Eye Health:

The vitamin A and antioxidants in melons promote vision health by supporting retinal function, reducing the risk of age-related macular degeneration, and protecting against cataracts.

Including melons in the diet may help maintain visual acuity and prevent eye disorders associated with aging.

Skin Health:

The vitamin C and antioxidants in melons promote collagen synthesis, reduce oxidative damage, and maintain skin elasticity and hydration.

Consuming melons may help prevent skin disorders, reduce the appearance of wrinkles and fine lines, and promote a healthy complexion.

Digestive Health:

The dietary fiber in melons promotes regular bowel movements, prevents constipation, and supports digestive health.

Melons contain enzymes such as bromelain and papain, which aid in the digestion of proteins and may help alleviate symptoms of indigestion and bloating.

Weight Management:

Melons are low in calories and high in water and dietary fiber, making them a filling and nutritious food choice for individuals seeking to manage their weight.

Incorporating melons into meals and snacks can help increase satiety, reduce calorie intake, and support weight loss and weight maintenance efforts.

Cooking Tips and Considerations:

Melons are incredibly versatile fruits that can be enjoyed in a variety of ways. Here are some tips for incorporating melons into your diet:

Fresh Consumption: Enjoy melons fresh and ripe on their own as a refreshing snack, or add them to fruit salads, smoothies, or yogurt parfaits for added flavor and nutrition.

Juicing: Blend melons into fresh juices or smoothies for a hydrating and nutritious beverage option. Combine melons with other fruits, vegetables, and herbs for unique flavor combinations.

Salads: Add diced or cubed melons to green salads, grain salads, or pasta salads for a sweet and juicy burst of flavor. Melons pair well with leafy greens, nuts, seeds, and cheese in salad recipes.

Appetizers and Starters: Use melons as a base for appetizers such as fruit skewers, bruschetta, or crostini, topped with savory or sweet ingredients for contrast.

Desserts: Incorporate melons into desserts such as sorbets, granitas, popsicles, or fruit tarts for a light and refreshing treat. Melons can also be grilled or caramelized for added depth of flavor.

Oats

A cup of oatmeal or oat bran has only 110 calories. And oats help you lose weight. Subjects in Dr. James Anderson's landmark 12-year study at the University of Kentucky lost three pounds in two months simply by adding 100 grams (3.5 ounces) of oat bran to their daily food intake and nothing else. Just don't expect oats alone to perform miracles – you have to eat a balanced diet for total health.

Nutritional Composition:

Oats are packed with essential nutrients, including complex carbohydrates, fiber, protein, vitamins, minerals, and antioxidants. A single serving of oats (approximately one cup cooked) typically contains the following nutrients:

Carbohydrates: Oats are a rich source of complex carbohydrates, providing sustained energy and promoting feelings of fullness and satiety. The complex carbohydrates in oats are digested slowly, resulting in a gradual release of glucose into the bloodstream and stable energy levels.

Fiber: Oats are exceptionally high in dietary fiber, containing both soluble and insoluble fibers. Soluble fiber, particularly beta-glucan, forms a gel-like substance in the digestive tract, which helps lower cholesterol levels, regulate blood sugar levels, and promote digestive health. Insoluble fiber adds bulk to stools, promotes regular bowel movements, and prevents constipation.

Protein: Oats are a good source of plant-based protein, containing all essential amino acids necessary for muscle repair, growth, and maintenance. Protein is also crucial for various physiological functions, including enzyme production, hormone regulation, and immune function.

Vitamins: Oats provide essential vitamins such as vitamin B1 (thiamine), vitamin B5 (pantothenic acid), and vitamin B6 (pyridoxine). These B vitamins play key roles in energy metabolism, nerve function, and red blood cell production. Oats also contain small amounts of vitamin E, a powerful antioxidant that protects cells from oxidative damage.

Minerals: Oats are rich in minerals such as manganese, phosphorus, magnesium, and zinc. Manganese is essential for bone formation, carbohydrate metabolism, and antioxidant defense. Phosphorus is necessary for bone health, energy production, and cell signaling. Magnesium supports muscle function, nerve transmission, and blood pressure regulation. Zinc is vital for immune function, wound healing, and protein synthesis.

Antioxidants: Oats contain various antioxidants, including avenanthramides and phenolic compounds, which help reduce inflammation, protect against oxidative stress, and lower the risk of chronic diseases such as heart disease, cancer, and diabetes.

Health Benefits:

Heart Health:

The soluble fiber beta-glucan in oats helps lower LDL (bad) cholesterol levels by reducing cholesterol absorption in the intestines and promoting bile acid excretion.

Regular consumption of oats is associated with a reduced risk of heart disease, stroke, and other cardiovascular conditions.

Blood Sugar Control:

The soluble fiber in oats slows down the digestion and absorption of carbohydrates, which helps regulate blood sugar levels and prevent spikes in insulin release.

Including oats in meals may help improve insulin sensitivity, reduce the risk of type 2 diabetes, and manage blood glucose levels in individuals with diabetes.

Digestive Health:

The high fiber content in oats promotes digestive health by preventing constipation, regulating bowel movements, and supporting a healthy gut microbiome.

Oats may help alleviate symptoms of gastrointestinal disorders such as irritable bowel syndrome (IBS) and diverticulosis.

Weight Management:

The combination of fiber, protein, and complex carbohydrates in oats promotes feelings of fullness and satiety, which can help control appetite and reduce calorie intake.

Including oats in meals and snacks may support weight loss and weight management efforts by preventing overeating and reducing cravings for high-calorie foods.

Improved Athletic Performance:

Oats are a popular choice among athletes and fitness enthusiasts due to their high carbohydrate content, which provides a readily available source of energy for exercise.

The protein in oats supports muscle recovery and repair, while the fiber helps maintain digestive health and prevent gastrointestinal discomfort during physical activity.

Lower Risk of Chronic Diseases:

The antioxidants and phytochemicals in oats help reduce inflammation, neutralize free radicals, and protect against oxidative damage, lowering the risk of chronic diseases such as cancer, Alzheimer's disease, and arthritis.

Including oats as part of a balanced diet rich in fruits, vegetables, whole grains, and lean proteins may help promote overall health and well-being.

Cooking Tips and Considerations:

Incorporating oats into your diet is simple and versatile, offering endless culinary possibilities. Here are some tips for enjoying oats:

Oatmeal: Cook oats with water or milk to make a hearty and nutritious breakfast porridge. Customize your oatmeal with toppings such as fresh fruits, nuts, seeds, and spices for added flavor and texture.

Overnight Oats: Prepare overnight oats by soaking rolled oats in milk or yogurt overnight, then topping them with your favorite fruits, nuts, and sweeteners for a convenient grab-and-go breakfast option.

Baking: Use oats in baking recipes such as cookies, muffins, bread, and granola bars to add texture, fiber, and nutritional value. Replace a portion of flour with oats in recipes to boost their fiber content.

Smoothies: Blend oats into smoothies or shakes for added thickness, creaminess, and nutritional value. Rolled oats or oat flour can be added to fruit-based or protein-rich smoothie recipes for a satisfying and filling beverage.

Savory Dishes: Use oats as a binding agent or thickener in savory dishes such as veggie burgers, meatloaf, soups, and stews. Rolled oats or oat flour can replace breadcrumbs or flour in recipes to create gluten-free alternatives.

Onions

Flavorful, aromatic, inexpensive, and low in calories, onions deserve a regular place in your diet. One cup of chopped raw onions has only 60 calories, and one raw medium onion (2.15" diameter) has just 42.

They control cholesterol, thin the blood, protect against cholesterol, and may have some value in counteracting allergic reactions. Most of all, onions taste good and they're good for you.

Partially boil, peel, and bake, basting with olive oil and lemon juice. Or sauté them in white wine and basil, then spread over pizza. Or roast them in sherry and serve over the paste.

Nutritional Profile:

Onions are low in calories yet rich in essential nutrients. A medium-sized onion typically contains:

Calories: 44

Carbohydrates: 10 grams

Fiber: 2 grams

Vitamin C: 12% of the Daily Value (DV)

Vitamin B6: 9% of the DV

Folate: 8% of the DV

Potassium: 5% of the DV

Additionally, onions are a good source of antioxidants, particularly quercetin and sulfur compounds, which contribute significantly to their health-promoting properties.

Antioxidant Properties:

Quercetin, a flavonoid abundant in onions, exhibits potent antioxidant activity. Antioxidants help neutralize free radicals, unstable molecules that can damage cells and contribute to chronic diseases such as cancer and cardiovascular ailments. Regular consumption of onions may thus confer protection against oxidative stress and reduce the risk of chronic illnesses.

Anti-Inflammatory Effects:

Sulfur compounds present in onions, including thiosulfinates and cepaenes, possess anti-inflammatory properties. These compounds inhibit the activity of inflammatory enzymes and cytokines, thereby alleviating inflammation throughout the body. Incorporating onions into the diet may help mitigate symptoms of inflammatory conditions such as arthritis and inflammatory bowel disease.

Heart Health Benefits:

Onions offer several cardiovascular benefits, primarily attributed to their antioxidant and anti-inflammatory properties. Quercetin, in particular, has been shown to lower blood pressure and reduce cholesterol levels, thereby decreasing the risk of heart disease. Furthermore, onions contain sulfur compounds that promote blood vessel dilation and inhibit platelet aggregation, reducing the likelihood of blood clots and improving circulation.

Cancer Prevention:

Epidemiological studies suggest that regular onion consumption may lower the risk of certain types of cancer, including colorectal, stomach, and prostate cancers. Quercetin and other phytochemicals found in onions exhibit anticancer properties by inhibiting tumor growth, inducing apoptosis (programmed cell death), and suppressing angiogenesis (the formation of new blood vessels to support tumor growth). While more research is needed to elucidate the precise mechanisms involved, incorporating onions into a balanced diet may contribute to cancer prevention strategies.

Immune Support:

The immune-boosting properties of onions can be attributed to their rich content of vitamin C and other immune-supportive nutrients. Vitamin C stimulates the production and function of white blood cells, the frontline defenders of the immune system. Additionally, the sulfur compounds in onions exhibit antimicrobial activity, helping fend off pathogens and reduce the severity of infections such as colds and flu.

Digestive Health:

Onions contain a type of fiber called fructooligosaccharides (FOS), which serves as a prebiotic, nourishing beneficial gut bacteria. By promoting the growth of probiotic bacteria in the intestines, FOS contributes to digestive health and helps maintain a balanced microbiome. Furthermore, the anti-inflammatory properties of onions may alleviate symptoms of gastrointestinal disorders such as gastritis and acid reflux.

Blood Sugar Regulation:

Despite their natural sweetness, onions have a low glycemic index (GI), meaning they have a minimal impact on blood sugar levels. This makes them suitable for individuals with diabetes or those aiming to manage their blood sugar levels. Moreover, certain compounds in onions, such as allyl propyl disulfide (APDS), have been shown to enhance insulin sensitivity, potentially reducing the risk of insulin resistance and type 2 diabetes.

Bone Health:

Onions contain several nutrients that are essential for maintaining strong and healthy bones, including calcium, magnesium, and vitamin C. These nutrients play crucial roles in bone formation, mineralization, and maintenance of bone density. Regular consumption of onions, along with other bone-supportive foods, may help prevent osteoporosis and reduce the risk of fractures, especially in aging populations.

Skin and Hair Benefits:

The antioxidants and sulfur compounds in onions offer various benefits for skin and hair health. Quercetin and other flavonoids help protect the skin from oxidative damage caused by environmental factors such as UV radiation and pollution, thus reducing the risk of premature aging and skin disorders. Moreover, sulfur compounds contribute to the production of collagen and keratin, proteins essential for maintaining the strength, elasticity, and luster of hair and nails.

Pasta

The Italians had it right all along. A cup of cooked paste (without a heavy sauce) has only 155 calories and fits the description of a perfect starch-centered staple. Analysis at the American Institute of Baking shows pasta is rich in six minerals, including manganese, iron, phosphorus, copper, magnesium and zinc. Also be sure to consider whole wheat pastas, which are even healthier.

Nutritional Composition:

Pasta serves as an excellent source of complex carbohydrates, providing sustained energy to fuel daily activities. A typical serving of cooked pasta (approximately 2 ounces or 56 grams) contains:

Calories: 200

Carbohydrates: 40 grams

Protein: 7 grams

Fiber: 2 grams

Fat: 1 gram

Various vitamins and minerals, including folate, iron, and magnesium.

Furthermore, pasta is low in sodium and cholesterol-free, making it a heart-healthy choice when prepared with wholesome ingredients.

Satiety and Weight Management:

Despite its reputation as a high-carbohydrate food, pasta can be a valuable ally in weight management when consumed in moderation and as part of a balanced diet. Its combination of complex carbohydrates and protein promotes satiety, helping to curb hunger and prevent overeating. Additionally, the fiber content in pasta contributes to a feeling of fullness and aids in digestion, potentially reducing overall calorie intake and supporting weight loss efforts.

Energy Source for Active Lifestyles:

Pasta's complex carbohydrates provide a steady and reliable source of energy, making it an ideal choice for athletes and individuals with active lifestyles. Whether fueling a pre-workout meal or replenishing glycogen stores post-exercise, pasta delivers the sustained energy needed to power through physical activities effectively. When paired with lean proteins and vegetables, pasta forms a balanced meal that supports muscle recovery and overall performance.

Heart Health Benefits:

Contrary to popular belief, pasta can be part of a heart-healthy diet when prepared with wholesome ingredients and enjoyed in moderation. Whole-grain pasta varieties, in particular, offer cardiovascular benefits due to their higher fiber content and lower glycemic index compared to refined pasta. Fiber helps lower cholesterol levels, regulate blood sugar, and promote healthy digestion, thereby reducing the risk of heart disease and improving overall cardiovascular health.

Blood Sugar Regulation:

The complex carbohydrates in pasta are digested more slowly than simple sugars, resulting in a gradual and steady release of glucose into the bloodstream. This slow digestion rate helps prevent rapid spikes and crashes in blood sugar levels, making pasta a suitable choice for individuals with diabetes or those aiming to manage their blood sugar levels. Pairing pasta with fiber-rich vegetables and lean proteins can further enhance its glycemic response and promote stable blood sugar control.

Nutrient Density and Versatility:

Pasta serves as a versatile canvas for incorporating a wide array of nutrient-dense ingredients, including vegetables, lean proteins, healthy fats, herbs, and spices. By pairing pasta with nutrient-rich accompaniments such as tomatoes, spinach, salmon, olive oil, and garlic, you can create delicious and wholesome meals that deliver a spectrum of essential vitamins, minerals, and antioxidants. Additionally, pasta dishes can be customized to accommodate various dietary preferences and restrictions, making them suitable for individuals following vegetarian, vegan, gluten-free, or dairy-free diets.

Culinary Diversity and Cultural Heritage:

Beyond its nutritional virtues, pasta embodies a rich tapestry of culinary diversity and cultural heritage. From the iconic spaghetti and meatballs of Italian-American cuisine to the delicate ravioli of Northern Italy, pasta comes in countless shapes, sizes, and preparations, each reflecting the traditions and flavors of its respective region. Exploring the world of pasta opens doors to a vast repertoire of recipes, techniques, and culinary experiences, inviting you to embark on a flavorful journey across continents and centuries.

Sweet Potatoes

You can make a meal out of them and not worry about gaining a pound – and you sure won't walk away from the table feeling hungry. Each sweet potato has about 103 calories. Their creamy orange flesh is one of the best sources of vitamin A you can consume.

You can bake, steam, or microwave them. Or add them to casseroles, soups, and many other dishes. Flavor with lemon juice or vegetable broth instead of butter.

Nutrient Profile:

Sweet potatoes are nutritional powerhouses, packed with an impressive array of vitamins, minerals, and antioxidants. A medium-sized sweet potato (about 5 inches long) typically contains:

Calories: 103

Carbohydrates: 24 grams

Fiber: 4 grams

Protein: 2 grams

Fat: 0 grams

Vitamin A: 438% of the Daily Value (DV)

Vitamin C: 37% of the DV

Vitamin B6: 16% of the DV

Potassium: 15% of the DV

Manganese: 19% of the DV

Additionally, sweet potatoes are rich in antioxidants such as beta-carotene, which gives them their characteristic orange hue, as well as other phytonutrients like anthocyanins and polyphenols.

Antioxidant Powerhouse:

The abundance of antioxidants in sweet potatoes, particularly beta-carotene, plays a crucial role in protecting cells from oxidative damage caused by free radicals. These compounds help combat inflammation, neutralize harmful molecules, and reduce the risk of chronic diseases such as heart disease, cancer, and neurodegenerative disorders. Regular consumption of sweet potatoes can thus contribute to overall health and longevity.

Heart Health Benefits:

Sweet potatoes offer several cardiovascular benefits, thanks to their high potassium content and low sodium levels. Potassium helps regulate blood pressure by counteracting the effects of sodium and promoting vasodilation, thereby reducing the risk of hypertension and stroke. Additionally, the fiber and antioxidants in sweet potatoes contribute to lower cholesterol levels, improved blood vessel function, and reduced inflammation, all of which support heart health and reduce the risk of cardiovascular disease.

Blood Sugar Regulation:

Despite their natural sweetness, sweet potatoes have a relatively low glycemic index (GI), meaning they cause a gradual and steady increase in blood sugar levels compared to high-GI foods. This makes them suitable for individuals with diabetes or those aiming to manage their blood sugar levels. The fiber content in sweet potatoes further contributes to stable blood sugar control by slowing down the absorption of glucose and promoting satiety, helping to prevent spikes and crashes in blood sugar levels.

Digestive Health:

Sweet potatoes are an excellent source of dietary fiber, with both soluble and insoluble fibers that support digestive health. Fiber adds bulk to stool, promotes regularity, and prevents constipation, while also feeding beneficial gut bacteria and supporting a healthy microbiome. Moreover, the antioxidants and anti-inflammatory properties of sweet potatoes may alleviate symptoms of digestive disorders such as irritable bowel syndrome (IBS) and promote gut integrity and overall gastrointestinal wellness.

Immune Support:

The high vitamin A and vitamin C content in sweet potatoes makes them valuable allies in supporting a robust immune system. Vitamin A plays a crucial role in maintaining the integrity of mucous membranes, the body's first line of defense against pathogens, while vitamin C enhances the function of immune cells and promotes the production of antibodies. By incorporating sweet potatoes into your diet, you can fortify your immune defenses and reduce the risk of infections and illnesses.

Vision and Eye Health:

Beta-carotene, the precursor to vitamin A found abundantly in sweet potatoes, is essential for maintaining healthy vision and eye function. It helps protect the eyes from oxidative damage, reduces the risk of age-related macular degeneration (AMD) and cataracts, and promotes good night vision. Regular consumption of sweet potatoes can thus contribute to long-term eye health and preserve visual acuity as you age.

Skin and Hair Benefits:

The antioxidants and vitamins in sweet potatoes offer various benefits for skin and hair health. Beta-carotene, in particular, helps protect the skin from sun damage, promotes collagen production, and imparts a healthy glow. Additionally, vitamin C supports collagen synthesis and acts as an antioxidant, while vitamin E contributes to skin hydration and protects against oxidative stress.

Including sweet potatoes in your diet can therefore nourish your skin from within and promote lustrous hair and radiant complexion.

Weight Management:

Despite their relatively high carbohydrate content, sweet potatoes can be a valuable component of a weight management plan due to their low energy density and high fiber content. Fiber promotes satiety, reduces hunger, and prolongs feelings of fullness, helping to control calorie intake and prevent overeating. Furthermore, the complex carbohydrates in sweet potatoes provide sustained energy, making them an excellent choice for fueling workouts and maintaining energy levels throughout the day.

Tomatoes

A medium tomato (2.5" diameter) has only about 25 calories. These garden delights are low in fat and sodium, high in potassium, and rich in fiber.

A survey at Harvard Medical School found that the chances of dying of cancer are lowest among people who eat tomatoes (or strawberries) every week.

And don't overlook canned crushed, peeled, whole or stewed tomatoes. They make sauces, casseroles, and soups taste great while retaining their nutritional goodness and low-calorie status. Even plain old spaghetti sauce is a fat-burning bargain when served over pasta, so think about introducing tomatoes into your diet.

Nutrient Composition:

Tomatoes are low in calories yet bursting with essential nutrients. A medium-sized tomato (approximately 123 grams) typically contains:

Calories: 22

Carbohydrates: 5 grams

Fiber: 1.5 grams

Protein: 1 gram

Fat: 0.2 grams

Vitamin C: 28% of the Daily Value (DV)

Vitamin K: 9% of the DV

Potassium: 6% of the DV

Folate: 5% of the DV

Lycopene: A powerful antioxidant pigment responsible for the vibrant red color of tomatoes.

Additionally, tomatoes are rich in other antioxidants such as beta-carotene, lutein, and zeaxanthin, as well as vitamins A, B6, and E, making them a nutrient-dense addition to any diet.

Antioxidant Properties:

Tomatoes are renowned for their high antioxidant content, particularly lycopene, which is associated with numerous health benefits. Lycopene exhibits potent antioxidant activity, scavenging free radicals and protecting cells from oxidative damage. This antioxidant prowess helps reduce inflammation, lower the risk of chronic diseases such as heart disease and cancer, and promote overall health and longevity.

Heart Health Benefits:

Regular consumption of tomatoes has been linked to improved heart health due to their rich antioxidant content and other cardioprotective compounds. Lycopene, in particular, has been shown to lower levels of LDL cholesterol, the "bad" cholesterol implicated in heart disease, and reduce the risk of atherosclerosis and cardiovascular events. Furthermore, tomatoes contain potassium, a mineral that helps regulate blood pressure and promote cardiovascular function.

Cancer Prevention:

Tomatoes possess potent anticancer properties attributed to their high levels of antioxidants, particularly lycopene. Epidemiological studies suggest that individuals who consume diets rich in tomatoes and tomato-based products have a lower risk of certain types of cancer, including prostate, lung, stomach, and breast cancer. Lycopene and other phytonutrients in tomatoes inhibit cancer cell proliferation, induce apoptosis (cell death), and suppress tumor growth, making tomatoes a valuable ally in cancer prevention and treatment.

Eye Health:

The antioxidant compounds in tomatoes, including lycopene, beta-carotene, lutein, and zeaxanthin, play a crucial role in supporting eye health and vision. These compounds help protect the eyes from oxidative damage caused by UV radiation and other environmental factors, reducing the risk of age-related macular degeneration (AMD) and cataracts. Regular consumption of tomatoes and tomato-based products can thus help preserve visual acuity and promote long-term eye health.

Skin Protection:

Tomatoes offer benefits for skin health and protection against sun damage, thanks to their rich antioxidant content. Lycopene, in particular, helps neutralize free radicals generated by UV radiation, reducing the risk of sunburn, premature aging, and skin cancer. Additionally, the vitamins and minerals in tomatoes support collagen production, promote skin hydration, and improve overall skin texture and tone, enhancing the skin's natural radiance and resilience.

Weight Management:

Tomatoes are an excellent addition to a weight management plan due to their low calorie and high water content, as well as their fiber-rich composition. The combination of fiber and water in tomatoes promotes satiety, reduces hunger, and increases feelings of fullness, making them a satisfying and nourishing option for those looking to control calorie intake and manage weight. Moreover, the vitamins and minerals in tomatoes support metabolic function and energy production, further enhancing their role in weight management.

Digestive Health:

The fiber content in tomatoes supports digestive health by promoting regularity, preventing constipation, and supporting a healthy gut microbiome. Additionally, tomatoes contain compounds such as citric acid and malic acid, which stimulate gastric secretion and aid in digestion. Consuming tomatoes as part of a balanced diet can thus contribute to digestive wellness and alleviate symptoms of digestive disorders such as bloating, indigestion, and irritable bowel syndrome (IBS).

Bone Health:

Tomatoes contain several nutrients essential for maintaining strong and healthy bones, including vitamin K, potassium, and calcium. Vitamin K plays a crucial role in bone mineralization and helps prevent osteoporosis, while potassium contributes to bone density and reduces the risk of bone fractures. Additionally, the antioxidant properties of tomatoes may help reduce inflammation and oxidative stress, which can contribute to bone loss and degenerative bone diseases.

Turkey

Give thanks to those pilgrims for starting the wonderful tradition of Thanksgiving turkey. It just so happens that this healthy food disguised as meat is good year-round for weight control.

A four-ounce serving of roasted white meat turkey has 177 calories and dark meat has 211.

Sadly, many folks are still unaware of the versatility and flavor of ground turkey. Anything hamburger can do, ground turkey can do at least as well, from conventional burgers to spaghetti sauce to meatloaf.

Some ground turkey contains skin which slightly increases the fat content. If you want to keep it lean, opt for ground-breasted meat. But since this has no added fat, you'll need to add filler to make burgers or meatloaf hold together.

Four ounces of ground turkey has approximately 170 calories and nine grams of fat – about what you'd find in 2.5 teaspoons of butter or margarine. Incredibly, the same amount of regular ground beef (21% fat) has 298 calories and 23 grams of fat.

Buying turkey has become easy. It's no longer necessary to buy a whole bird unless you want to. Ground turkey is available fresh or frozen, as are individual parts of the bird, including drumsticks, thighs, breasts, and cutlets.

Nutrient Profile:

Turkey is prized for its lean meat, which is low in fat yet packed with essential nutrients. A 3-ounce (85-gram) serving of roasted turkey breast typically contains:

Calories: 135

Protein: 26 grams

Fat: 3 grams

Iron: 2% of the Daily Value (DV)

Zinc: 8% of the DV

Phosphorus: 14% of the DV

Selenium: 30% of the DV

Vitamin B6: 20% of the DV

Vitamin B12: 10% of the DV

Niacin: 40% of the DV

Additionally, turkey is a good source of other vitamins and minerals, including potassium, magnesium, and riboflavin.

High-Quality Protein:

Turkey stands out as an excellent source of high-quality protein, containing all the essential amino acids needed for muscle growth, repair, and maintenance. Protein plays a crucial role in supporting various bodily functions, including enzyme production, hormone regulation, and immune function. Incorporating turkey into your diet can help meet your daily protein needs and promote muscle health, satiety, and overall well-being.

Weight Management:

Despite its rich flavor and satisfying texture, turkey is relatively low in calories and fat, making it an ideal choice for individuals looking to manage their weight or maintain a healthy body composition. The high protein content of turkey helps promote satiety, reduce hunger, and control appetite, leading to fewer calories consumed overall. Furthermore, protein-rich foods like turkey have a higher thermic effect, meaning they require more energy to digest and metabolize, potentially enhancing calorie expenditure and supporting weight loss efforts.

Heart Health Benefits:

Turkey offers several cardiovascular benefits, primarily attributed to its lean protein content and low saturated fat levels. Diets rich in lean protein sources like turkey have been associated with improved cholesterol profiles, reduced blood pressure, and decreased risk of heart disease. Additionally, turkey contains nutrients such as selenium and B vitamins, which support heart health by reducing inflammation, preventing oxidative stress, and promoting proper cardiovascular function.

Immune Support:

The nutrients in turkey, including zinc, selenium, and vitamin B6, play essential roles in supporting immune function and strengthening the body's defenses against infections and illnesses. Zinc and selenium act as antioxidants, helping neutralize free radicals and protect immune cells from damage. Vitamin B6, on the other hand, supports the production of immune cells and antibodies, enhancing the body's ability to fight off pathogens. Including turkey in your diet can thus bolster your immune system and promote overall resilience to infections.

Muscle Health and Exercise Performance:

As a rich source of high-quality protein, turkey is particularly beneficial for individuals engaged in regular physical activity or strength training. Protein is essential for muscle repair and growth, helping to rebuild and strengthen muscle fibers damaged during exercise. Consuming turkey post-workout can facilitate muscle recovery, reduce soreness, and promote optimal exercise performance. Additionally, the amino acid leucine, abundant in turkey protein, plays a key role in stimulating muscle protein synthesis, further supporting muscle health and adaptation to exercise.

Mood Regulation:

Turkey contains nutrients that play vital roles in neurotransmitter synthesis and mood regulation, including tryptophan, vitamin B6, and folate. Tryptophan is a precursor to serotonin, a neurotransmitter involved in mood regulation, sleep, and appetite control. Vitamin B6 and folate contribute to the synthesis and metabolism of neurotransmitters, supporting proper brain function and emotional well-being. Incorporating turkey into your diet can thus help maintain stable mood levels, reduce stress, and support overall mental health.

Hair and Skin Health:

The nutrients in turkey, including protein, zinc, and B vitamins, are essential for maintaining healthy hair and skin. Protein provides the building blocks for strong and resilient hair and skin tissues, while zinc supports collagen synthesis and promotes wound healing. B vitamins such as biotin and niacin contribute to hair growth, texture, and shine, as well as skin hydration and elasticity. Including turkey in your diet can thus nourish your hair and skin from within, promoting lustrous locks and a radiant complexion.

Yogurt

The non-fat variety of plain yogurt has 120 calories per cup and low-fat, 144. It delivers a lot of protein and, like any dairy food, is rich in calcium and contains zinc and riboflavin.

Yogurt is handy as a breakfast food – cut a banana into it and add the cereal of your choice.

You can find ways to use it in other types of cooking, to – sauces, soups, dips, toppings, stuffings, and spreads. Many kitchen gadget departments even sell a simple funnel for making yogurt cheese.

Yogurt can replace heavy creams and whole milk in a wide range of dishes, saving scads of fat and calories.

You can substitute half or all of the higher-fat ingredients. Be creative. For example, combine yogurt, garlic powder, lemon juice, a dash of pepper, and Worcestershire sauce and use it to top a baked potato instead of piling on fat-laden sour cream.

Supermarkets and health food stores sell a variety of yogurts, many with added fruit and sugar. To control calories and fat content, buy plain non-fat yogurt and add fruit yourself. Apple butter or fruit spreads with little or no added sugar are an excellent way to turn plain yogurt into a delectable sweet treat.

Nutrient-Rich Composition:

Yogurt is a nutritional powerhouse, packed with essential nutrients that contribute to overall health and vitality. A typical serving of yogurt (about 6 ounces or 170 grams) contains:

Calories: 150

Protein: 12 grams

Carbohydrates: 17 grams

Fat: 5 grams

Calcium: 30% of the Daily Value (DV)

Vitamin B12: 22% of the DV

Riboflavin (Vitamin B2): 20% of the DV

Phosphorus: 20% of the DV

Potassium: 11% of the DV

Probiotics: Live beneficial bacteria that promote gut health.

Additionally, yogurt is a good source of other vitamins and minerals, including vitamin D, magnesium, and zinc, making it a nutrient-dense addition to any diet.

Probiotic Content:

One of the most significant health benefits of yogurt lies in its probiotic content. Probiotics are live beneficial bacteria that confer various health advantages when consumed in adequate amounts. Yogurt contains strains of probiotic bacteria such as Lactobacillus acidophilus, Lactobacillus bulgaricus, and Bifidobacterium lactis, which promote gut health, support digestion, and strengthen the immune system. Regular consumption of yogurt can help maintain a healthy balance of gut microbiota and alleviate symptoms of digestive disorders such as bloating, gas, and diarrhea.

Digestive Health:

Yogurt is renowned for its ability to promote digestive health and alleviate symptoms of gastrointestinal discomfort. The probiotic bacteria in yogurt help regulate bowel movements, improve nutrient absorption, and maintain intestinal barrier function. Additionally, yogurt contains lactase, an enzyme that aids in the digestion of lactose, making it suitable for individuals with lactose intolerance. Incorporating yogurt into your diet can thus support optimal digestion, reduce digestive distress, and promote overall gastrointestinal wellness.

Immune Support:

The probiotics in yogurt play a crucial role in supporting immune function and strengthening the body's defenses against infections and illnesses. Probiotic bacteria help modulate the immune response, stimulate the production of immune cells and antibodies, and enhance the gut-brain axis, which regulates immune function and inflammatory responses. Consuming yogurt regularly can thus bolster the immune system, reduce the risk of respiratory infections, and promote overall resilience to diseases.

Bone Health:

Yogurt is a rich source of calcium, a mineral essential for maintaining strong and healthy bones. Adequate calcium intake is crucial for bone mineralization, density, and strength, helping prevent osteoporosis and reduce the risk of fractures and bone disorders. Additionally, yogurt contains protein and other nutrients such as phosphorus, magnesium, and vitamin D, which further support bone health and contribute to overall skeletal integrity. Including yogurt in your diet can thus help meet your daily calcium needs and promote lifelong bone health.

Weight Management:

Despite its creamy texture and rich flavor, yogurt can be a valuable ally in weight management when consumed as part of a balanced diet. The protein and probiotics in yogurt promote satiety, reduce appetite, and prolong feelings of fullness, making it an excellent option for controlling calorie intake and managing hunger. Additionally, yogurt contains conjugated linoleic acid (CLA), a type of fatty acid that may help reduce body fat accumulation and promote weight loss. Choosing plain yogurt with no added sugars and incorporating it into meals and snacks can support healthy weight management goals.

Cardiovascular Health:

Emerging research suggests that yogurt consumption may have favorable effects on cardiovascular health, including reducing the risk of heart disease and stroke. The calcium, potassium, and magnesium in yogurt help regulate blood pressure, promote vasodilation, and maintain proper cardiac function. Furthermore, the probiotics in yogurt may improve lipid profiles by reducing levels of LDL cholesterol (the "bad" cholesterol) and triglycerides while increasing levels of HDL cholesterol (the "good" cholesterol). Enjoying yogurt as part of a heart-healthy diet may thus contribute to overall cardiovascular wellness and reduce the risk of cardiovascular diseases.

Skin and Hair Benefits:

The nutrients in yogurt, including protein, vitamins, and minerals, offer various benefits for skin and hair health. Protein supports collagen synthesis, helping maintain skin elasticity and firmness, while vitamins such as riboflavin and vitamin B12 promote cell regeneration and repair. Additionally, the lactic acid in yogurt acts as a gentle exfoliant, removing dead skin cells and impurities, and promoting a smoother and more radiant complexion. Furthermore, yogurt can be used topically as a natural hair conditioner and moisturizer, thanks to its nourishing properties. Incorporating yogurt into your diet and skincare routine can thus enhance the health and appearance of your skin and hair.